ACCIDENTAL WEIGHT LOSS

8 Hidden Secrets For Losing Weight Without Even Trying

JEREMY HENDON

J&L Publishing LLC.

TABLE OF CONTENTS

THE BUILDING BLOCKS OF WEIGHT LOSS

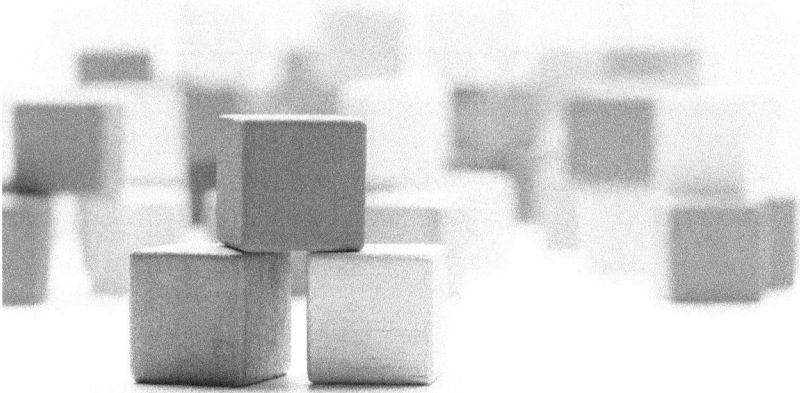

IN 1878, AFTER a short business trip, Milton Wright returned home to Cedar Rapids, Iowa.

As a gift for his children, he brought back a toy made of paper and bamboo. The toy—when twisted with a rubber band—would fly through the air. Here's a sketch of what that toy looked like . . .

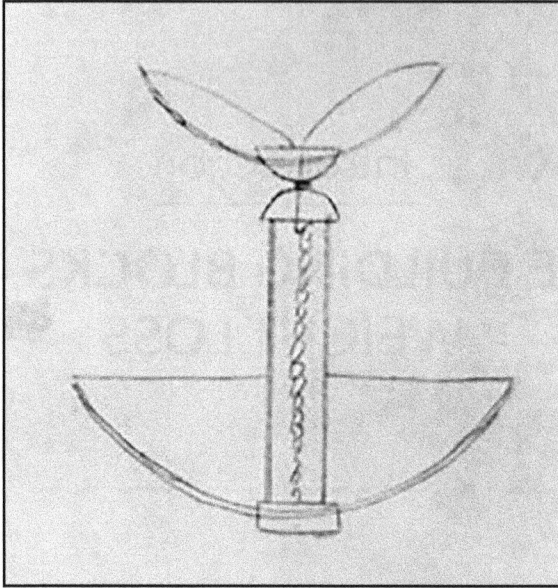

Two of his sons, Will and Orv, loved the toy and started playing with it all the time. Much later, they told a reporter that the toy was a big inspiration for them to eventually build and fly the first controlled, human-powered aircraft.

They were, of course, the Wright Brothers, Wilbur and Orville.

However, their dad bought the toy when they were 7 and 11 years old, and it wasn't until 25 years later that they finally flew their first airplane. Why was that the case, and what happened in between?

As I'll show you, the life story of the Wright Brothers' is not *just* a great story.

The story of the Wright Brothers holds the secret to losing weight, breaking through plateaus, and finally looking in the mirror and being happy with your body.

But before I tell you the rest of the story, you should answer 3 questions for yourself . . .

3 Important Questions for You

1. Is losing weight something that is *deeply* important to you and that will make a *real* difference in your life?

2. Have you tried to lose weight, but you've either failed or stalled in your weight loss? (Or maybe you've even regained some of the weight you lost?)

3. Are you open to trying a better way of losing weight, even if it means un-learning some of what you've been taught?

If you can answer YES to all 3 of these questions, then I've written this book specifically for you, and you're likely to get great results (although nothing is ever guaranteed in health).

If losing weight and getting healthy are *deeply important* to you, then this book has the potential to dramatically change and improve your life. And if you're open to doing things a *little bit differently*, then you're in the right place.

In this book, I'm going to show you a simpler and more sustainable way of losing weight. But I won't lie—it will require a little bit of work and determination from you.

After all, the Wright Brothers didn't sit around for 25 years before they built and flew their first plane . . .

The Long and Winding Road

In 1889, Orville Wright dropped out of high school and founded a printing company with Wilbur. They didn't have money to buy a printing press machine, so they built their own from "a damaged tombstone, buggy parts, and other recycled odds and ends."

Within a couple years, the company was a success, and they upgraded to a larger and better printing press.

Then, in 1892, bicycles started getting very popular across the country. So Wilbur and Orville changed direction and opened a bicycle repair shop.

Within another couple of years, they were manufacturing and selling their own brand of bikes. The brothers built custom bikes for customers, and they also invented several improvements to bikes (such as coaster brakes) that are still used 120 years later.

As a result, the bike business was very successful and profitable, which provided the brothers with a substantial amount of money.

Throughout both the printing business and the bicycle business, Wilbur and Orville learned and mastered every skill they needed to succeed. They mastered the skills of building a faster printing press, installing coaster brakes on bikes, and even learning to sell and advertise their services.

And after mastering one skill, they would simply move on to another skill, all in an effort to improve their machines, their products, and themselves.

The Promised Land

In 1898, the brothers began to get serious about aeronautics.

Many people were attempting to fly, but three big problems were holding everyone back:

- Engines were either too heavy or not powerful enough.
- Wings didn't have enough lift.
- Aircrafts couldn't be controlled well (turning, banking, etc.).

The Wright brothers knew they needed to solve all three problems, but they decided to tackle the most important one first: lack of control.

Wilbur and Orville believed that flying was just like riding a bike, only up in the sky. So like a bike, they wanted the pilot to have absolute control over the plane. (This sounds obvious now, but at the time, it was not the most popular approach.)

While in the bike shop, Wilbur tested the idea of twisting the wings (called "wing-warping")—an idea he got from randomly twisting a box in the bike shop in the same way that a bird's wings would twist. And the idea was a good one.

By 1900, they had successfully tested many kites and gliders with this "wing-warping" technology. So they started looking for the perfect location to test a glider *with a passenger*. In order to successfully fly a glider, you need two things that aren't found in Ohio: soft landing surfaces and the proper wind.

So, they ended up in Kitty Hawk, North Carolina.

From 1900 until 1903, the brothers tested countless gliders, making tweaks to *everything*. They used a bike wheel to test drag on the wings, they tested various angles of wings, and they crashed <u>hundreds of times</u>.

However, in December of 1903, in front of 5 observers, the brothers finally flew their aircraft four different times, at distances of 120 feet, 175 feet, 200 feet, and 852 feet. Seven years later, they took their father—who'd originally brought them home the flying toy—on his first flight.

You can imagine how <u>proud</u> Wilbur and Orville must have felt.

The Wright Brothers became American icons, and everybody now knows their names. But why should any of this be important to you?

Most importantly, how can their story help <u>you</u> lose weight?

<u>Weight Loss is a LOT Like Flying</u>

The Wright Brothers were intelligent, patient, and persistent.

But none of those qualities were the *real* reasons that they were the first people to build and fly an airplane.

And this is also true of weight loss. It doesn't matter how smart you are, for instance. You probably know people who are brilliant but can't seem to lose weight. You might be one of those people.

For the Wright Brothers, there were *2 Keys* to their success at flying.

And although it might not seem obvious, <u>these are the same keys that can help you to lose weight and get healthier</u>. In fact, these are the 2 keys for doing well at anything in life.

After all, very few people are able to lose weight and keep it off, just like very few people were able to build and fly a plane.

I want to share these 2 keys with you, and then I'll explain why they matter so much for weight loss . . .

Success Key #1: Mastering the Fundamentals (All of Them)

Wilbur and Orville mastered *every* fundamental skill they needed to fly a plane. And they solved *every* problem that blocked their path.

- They learned how to build and operate machines in their printing business.

- They learned to repair and build vehicles (bikes). And they used many of the same (bicycle) parts to build their first planes.

- In their bicycle business, they raised enough money to fund their planes.

- They relocated to a location (North Carolina) with ideal winds, hills, and landing areas.

- They learned to control an aircraft by watching birds fly and then modeling the movement of the bird's wings with a bike tube box.

- Through hundreds of test flights, they mastered building gliders with proper wing angles and wingspan.

And that's just a *short list* of the fundamental skills they mastered and the problems they solved.

Wilbur and Orville had to overcome a LOT to become the first humans to fly.

Luckily, **mastering the fundamentals of weight loss is far easier than mastering the fundamentals of flying or many other endeavors**. And best of all, to see results in weight loss, you won't need to master 100% of the fundamentals.

Years later, the Wright Brothers remarked that they were *lucky* and that if it happened all over again, they probably wouldn't succeed. That's not actually true. It wasn't *lucky* that they built and flew the first airplane to be flown by humans.

They succeeded as <u>an accident</u> of doing all the right things—of mastering the fundamentals.

As it turns out, every success in history—from athletes to scientists—is the same kind of accident. Success is about getting ***all the pieces*** to line up so that everything ***suddenly*** clicks into place. Your ability to lose weight and get healthy is no exception.

I'll show you later in this book exactly what the fundamentals of weight loss are. In addition, I'll show you why they're easier to master, even if you don't feel that way right now. The truth is that the fundamentals of weight loss are already built into your body, and all you need to do is allow those fundamentals to come out.

But there's also a second key . . .

Success Key #2: One-Step-At-A-Time

The Wright Brothers developed their skills and knowledge over the course of their *25-year* journey.

They didn't wait until 1903 to try to earn enough money to build their planes. Nor did they wait 25 years to start learning about machines and aerodynamics. They learned and mastered all of these things one-at-a-time, over many years.

Don't worry—You don't need to spend 25 years trying to lose weight (although many people struggle for this long because they approach the problem in the wrong way).

The Wright Brothers learned about machines while operating their printing company. They learned basic mechanics and dynamics while building bikes. They earned money to fund their ventures through various businesses.

If they had tried to master every skill all at once, they would have ultimately failed. They wouldn't have had the time or knowledge to make any progress. And they would have been overwhelmed.

It's easy to look back at history and see what went right and wrong. But these lessons are just as applicable to weight-loss, dieting, and the current state of health.

2 Big Weight-Loss "Secrets" (Or Why All Diets Work Sometimes)

Have you ever noticed that there are as many diet books as there are stars in the sky?

If you read these books, most of them contain astounding success stories. Maybe you think that these stories are fake. And some of them might be.

But I know many authors of these books, and most of the success stories are real. So even though health and obesity are generally headed in the wrong direction, each of these diets is able to produce amazing results in at least <u>some</u> people.

How is that possible?

And why is it that no single diet seems to work for everybody? (Hint: Humans are all 99.9% the same, so it's not that every body is different.)

There are <u>2 "secrets"</u> why most diets work for some people but not for everybody. And these 2 secrets are very closely related to the Success Keys above . . .

Secret #1: All Good Diets Are Based on Some of the Same Fundamental Principles

Everybody tries to make their diet *seem* very different and very new. But the surprising truth is this . . .

Almost all modern diets are based on the <u>same 8 fundamental principles</u>.

If an author is trying to sell a lot of books, then he or she wants his or her diet to seem very unique.

But it's just not true. Paleo, Ketogenic, Mediterranean, Gluten-Free, Whole30, Virgin, Dash, and most other diets are more similar than different.

This is great news for you, because you don't need to try 20 different diets. All you need to do is apply the underlying fundamental principles. In this book, I'll call these fundamentals the "**8 Fundamental Principles of Effective Weight Loss**".

And in Chapter 4, I'll show you exactly what these fundamental principles are. They generally include basic things like removing inflammatory foods from your diet, automatically regulating hunger, and moving more.

However, very few diets get *all* of the fundamental principles right.

This is very important, so I'll write it again . . . **Most diets do NOT get all of the fundamental principles right—just a few.**

You would think that a diet book or expert would tell you everything you need to know in order to lose weight. But almost all diet books only tell you a *part* of what you need to know.

In other words, most diets emphasize just one or two principles.

That's why *some* people see success from *every* diet system. Even if a diet gets just one principle right, that might be exactly what somebody is missing.

For instance, a gluten-free diet book will tell you to stop eating wheat. And somebody in the world *needs* to hear only that particular advice. She might be doing everything else right (eating well, sleeping enough, exercising, etc.), but she might be very sensitive to wheat.

And if that person makes this one change, then she might get quickly healthier and lose weight.

Most diets get *some* principles right. But some is probably not enough for you, or else you would have already lost the weight you want to lose. You've got to know and apply all 8 principles. After all, you can't complete a puzzle if you only have 5 of the 8 pieces.

In addition, though . . .

Secret #2: All Diets Miss One Thing: The "Run then Rest" System

You've got to get the fundamental principles right to lose weight and be healthy. And yet, there's another piece that is at least as important.

If you're going to lose weight, you need to do what I call "Run then Rest."

Most diets make one of two mistakes:

- Some diets last for just a few weeks or months. They assume that you'll be fine after that, even if you go back to eating junk food and sitting on the couch; or

- Some diets assume that you'll keep going nonstop on the diet (forever).

Both of these mistakes will doom your diet and cause you to eventually regain any weight that you lose.

If you diet for a few weeks and then go back to eating junk food, you're going to regain any weight you lose. On the other hand, it's almost impossible to stick to a very restrictive diet for many years. Our human brains just aren't built to handle dieting forever.

For example, kids grow in spurts. They don't grow gradually, and they don't continue growing forever. Likewise, professional athletes train hard, but they also take days and weeks off.

Weight loss is no different. If you talk to anyone who's lost 100 or 200 pounds, they didn't do it all in one go, even if they *tried* to do it that way.

What actually happened was that they'd lose weight very well for a couple of months, then they'd stall for a little while, and then they'd repeat the cycle. There might be exceptions, but this is the rule for almost everyone who successfully loses a lot of weight.

So why don't all diets incorporate this fact into their diet from the beginning?

I can't answer for everybody, but it's probably because they want you to think weight loss is complicated and that they're the only ones with the answer. Or else, they don't actually know the answer.

The truth is that weight loss is not complicated. On the contrary . . .

Weight Loss is an Accident (But It's Not Luck)

Like being able to build the first plane, losing weight is also an accident—it's a side effect of being healthy and living a healthy lifestyle. In other words, **if you master the fundamentals of being healthy, you'll look great and lose weight by accident.**

You don't need to get lucky, and you can do it in a variety of ways. There's no particular food you need to eat, no specific exercise you need to do, and no expensive supplement you need to take.

But you do need to develop the skills and habits to be healthy. And just like the Wright Brothers, once you master these skills and habits, weight loss will *suddenly* happen *by accident*.

If you try to lose weight <u>without</u> being healthy, one of two things will happen: either (a) you won't succeed at all or (b) you'll gain back all the weight.

There is no gimmick or trick to losing weight. You've got to take care of your body and mind. Period.

And I know this not just from the people with whom I've worked, but also very deeply from my own experience, which I'll share with you in the next chapter.

This book will show you <u>exactly</u> how to *accidentally* lose weight.

I'll show you, step-by-step, all of the pieces of the puzzle. You might be missing one or you might be missing five.

It doesn't matter where you're starting. By implementing the "Big Wins" I'll show you, you can get from where you are now to your ideal body.

You'll likely see some quick results when you use this book. Many people do. But I believe that it's more important for you to be able to see *long-term results*.

And here's how to make that happen . . .

How to Get the Best Results for Your Body From This Book

I help folks lose weight and get healthy by mastering the fundamentals— the basics. And I help them do that by using "Dashes" and "Rests," which is the simplest and most powerful way to build a healthy life and a lean body.

This book is divided into 4 parts:

i. **<u>Part 1</u>** will show you why what you're doing now isn't working; it will also address some common myths and misconceptions. Part 1 will also cover the <u>8 Fundamental Principles of Effective Weight Loss</u>. These are the principles necessary for *accidental* and *sustained* weight loss.

ii. **Part 2** will show you the <u>Big Wins</u> in each area of your life (diet, exercise, etc.). These Big Wins are the easiest and most effective ways for you to implement the 8 Fundamental Principles and start losing weight by accident.

iii. **Part 3** covers the "Run then Rest" system and includes a Quick-Start Guide for implementing the system and starting to lose weight immediately.

iv. **Part 4** answers all of your questions and covers the most common mistakes that you can make.

I've tried to make this book as short as possible. You don't really need a lot of information. There's enough of that on the internet and in other books.

What you need is a system that has been proven to work over and over again. I'm only interested in what works, based on a lot of experience and results.

Feel free to use this book however you like. But remember, the basis of this book is getting Big Wins through the Run then Rest system. Part 2, in particular, contains a lot of information, and it might be tempting to try to do everything at once. If you do, you'll likely fail.

Remember . . . you've subjected your body to malnourishment and abuse for decades. You will likely see progress very quickly, but your body won't be able to heal itself in a week.

Most people who follow this system start to see results within a couple weeks. But more importantly, it's very likely that you'll start to feel better overall. You'll likely have more energy, be in a better mood, and also be able to think more clearly.

Some people have even told me that they've healed problems they forgot they had, because those problems had been part of their life for so long that they became the norm (such as cravings, mood swings, acne, IBS, autoimmune conditions, exhaustion, and insomnia). Amazing, huh?

Like anybody, I can't guarantee specific results or any results at all. But I can guarantee you that **what I've done is take the approaches from the most successful people in the world at losing weight and staying healthy**.

Finally, Let Me Know How it Goes

My biggest fear of writing any book is that it won't actually help anybody. I know for sure that the methods in this book work, and yet I still have this fear.

So if you do find success, please let me know. You can reach me at jeremy@jeremyhendon.com, and I absolutely love hearing from readers.

In addition, if you have any questions about the book, I'd also love to hear. I can't promise to have 100% of the answers, but if I don't, I usually know where to point somebody.

PART I

THE 8 FUNDAMENTAL PRINCIPLES OF EFFECTIVE WEIGHT LOSS

Chapter 1

A LIFETIME OF STRUGGLE

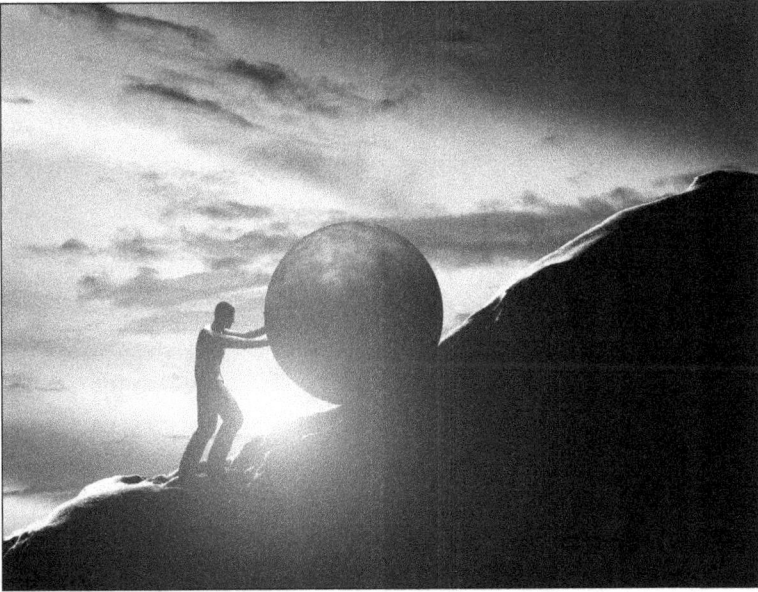

IF YOU'RE READING this book, I assume that you've struggled to lose weight.

Most people struggle for years, decades, or even their entire lives. And often, things get worse rather than getting better.

I've had many folks come to me who've gone from overweight to pre-diabetic to worse. And if you look around, it's not hard to see that things seem to be going in the wrong direction for most people.

I was one of those people . . .

I Personally Struggled My Whole Life with Being Overweight

I spent my entire life (from the time I was 6 years old) struggling with my weight. By the time I was 18, losing weight was an obsession for me.

It wasn't until my early 30s that I started to have consistent success at losing weight and keeping it off. And even then, it was extremely hard for me.

There are a few reasons why I'm telling you how hard it was for me— and it's not to make you feel bad for me:

1. First, I understand the struggle you're going through, both physically and emotionally. Being overweight was the thing I hated most about myself for a very long time, and even today, I'm still scared of gaining weight.

2. Second, because I've been obsessed with this for so long, I've tried dozens of different weight loss techniques, and I've read and researched a ridiculous amount about weight loss. I've also worked with, talked to, and interviewed hundreds of weight loss experts, from doctors to nutritionists to athletic coaches. I don't claim to be the world's leading expert on weight loss, but I'm excellent at finding what really works and helping people implement it.

3. Third—and most importantly—if I was able to finally lose weight and keep it off, then you can do it too. There are certainly folks who've had it tougher than me, but I've been through the wringer when it comes to weight loss.

In this book, I'm going to tell you **only** what's most important about weight loss, and I'm going to make it as simple as possible.

My only goal is to get you to actually **use** the information in this book to lose weight.

And here's where I want to begin . . .

I Spent a Lifetime Trying to Lose Weight in All the Wrong Ways

When I was 7 years old, I remember being upset that I couldn't run as fast or as long as the other kids on my basketball team.

By the time I was 9, I wouldn't take off my t-shirt at pool parties. I was too embarrassed of other kids seeing me without a shirt.

When I was 12, other kids threw rocks at me for a couple weeks on my way to my English class, all because (in their words) I was fat, walked funny, and hadn't ever had a girlfriend.

I've been insecure about the way I look for almost my entire life. And even though I'm much leaner now, I still carry that insecurity with me.

So when I got to college, my primary mission was to lose weight. I even enlisted my friend John to join me in a crusade to get in amazing shape.

At the time, pretty much everybody (the other kids in my dorm, relatives, and friends from high school) all told us that we shouldn't worry about losing weight and that doing it while in college was too tough. After all, most kids *gain* weight during their first year in college.

But we were determined, so we started doing the *obvious* things. We started running. We ate low-fat foods. And we played lots of sports.

There were many times that I wanted to give up (and there were times that John did), but I just kept going. I started running up to 60 miles per week and I kept eating what I thought was healthy (low-fat) food. After 9 months, I'd lost 55 pounds.

As you can probably imagine, I was very happy.

But like most weight loss stories, it didn't last. I injured my foot and stopped running. I eventually lost the willpower to eat only low-fat foods. And I gained pretty much all of the weight back.

For the next 10 years or so, I "yo-yo'd" back and forth between losing a bunch of weight and then gaining most of it back. In the process, I developed adrenal fatigue, hypothyroidism, and an unhealthy relationship with food.

It wasn't easy losing 55 pounds when I was 18 years old. It only got harder after that. Even after adopting a real-foods (Paleo) diet, losing weight and keeping it off wasn't as easy as I thought it should be.

I spent most of my life feeling like I was doing everything possible but nothing was working. And that is an incredibly discouraging way to feel.

But a few years ago, everything changed. It wasn't an immediate "aha" moment, and I didn't immediately discover the one trick I'd been missing all those years.

It gradually dawned on me, though, that I wasn't having trouble keeping the fat off any more. I wasn't struggling, I definitely wasn't starving myself or working out like a mad man, and everything just felt better and simpler.

The TWO THINGS I'd Been Missing All Those Years

After I thought for a long time about what was making everything easier for me, I finally figured it out.

The one thing I'd been missing was actually two things. (And I've already mentioned these things in the Introduction.)

1. EVERYTHING (The 8 Fundamental Principles). The first thing I had been missing was getting "everything" right.

Let me ask you a question . . .

What is necessary for a seed to sprout into a healthy plant?

Great soil? Plenty of sunlight? The right amount of water? Not too much competition? A perfect temperature range?

The correct answer is "yes."

It's all of those things. Without any one of them, the seed either won't sprout at all or else it will quickly die.

And that's the first thing I realized about my health and weight loss. It wasn't one thing that got me there or that made it all work out in the end. It was all the habits, systems, knowledge, and practices that I'd built up along the way.

By the time I realized that everything was working, I was eating a great diet, I was moving around enough, I wasn't as stressed as I used to be, and I'd cleaned up my gut—just to name a few.

If any one of those pieces of the puzzle hadn't been in place, then I likely would have continued to struggle. And if you're struggling right now, then you almost certainly don't have all pieces of the puzzle in place.

2. NOT ALL AT ONCE (The Run then Rest System). The second thing I'd been missing was ***not*** doing everything all at once.

I got lucky. I had simply been trying for so long that I'd finally gotten everything right. But it took me almost 20 years.

And during that 20 years, there were many times when I was very strict and focused. But there were also times when I "rested."

Let's be clear, though.

I didn't usually rest *intentionally*. It happened because I would run out of willpower. I'd cheat and then stop dieting or exercising for a while.

Then I'd try again, usually by focusing on something slightly different. But along the way, I kept building skills and habits that added up over time.

Obviously, the way I did it is not ideal. You don't want to wait 20 years for results.

Luckily, that's where I can help.

Completing the Puzzle

I haven't yet revealed the 8 Fundamental Principles of Effective Weight Loss, but I hope it makes sense why you need all of the puzzle pieces (diet, exercise, mindset, gut health, etc.) in order to lose weight.

Imagine if Orville and Wilbur Wright had never moved to Kitty Hawk and never had the proper winds to fly their plane. No matter what else they'd done right, they still wouldn't have been able to fly.

They needed to have all the puzzle pieces in place, just like you do in order to lose weight. But there's a twist to the story. Even though you need all of the puzzle pieces in place . . .

You Don't Need to Be Perfect!

The Wright Brothers needed good wind, they needed to model the wings after birds, and they needed to have the money to build multiple planes. But they didn't need to build a *perfect* plane. It didn't need rust-proof paint, jet propulsion, or 400 seats.

And in order to be healthy and lose weight, you also don't need to be perfect. You don't even need to eat a perfect diet.

But you *must* focus on what really matters for your particular goal.

For instance, if you want to lose weight, you don't really need to eat organic. Organic is great for health—it just doesn't matter very much for weight loss. It's the same reason that the Wright Brothers didn't paint their plane with rust-proof paint. It wasn't going to help it fly any better.

And that's just one example. Cardio, supplements, and avoiding GMOs are other examples. It's not that they're good or bad. They just don't matter for your particular goal.

I've seen countless people lose weight successfully, and I've talked to countless others who can't get it to work. People who successfully lose weight stay focused on the things that matter most.

The rest of this book will show you what really matters, and it will also show you how to incorporate it all into your life so that you can stick to it.

Getting One Thing Right is Not Usually Enough

Let me give you an example . . .

I love a real food or Paleo diet. I think it's one of the best ways to heal your body, to feel better than ever, and to lose weight.

But it's not always enough. And you probably know that already.

Diet is just one piece of the puzzle.

There are thousands of success stories of people losing weight. However, the failures don't get reported very often. You won't see a viral Facebook post about "How I Didn't Lose 30 Pounds in the Last 30 Days."

I've personally talked to hundreds of people who've had that experience. These people—just like you—see everyone around them getting results and losing weight, but it just doesn't work for them. And often, they feel like a failure for that reason.

If you're in that situation, then please understand that you have not failed.

All that it means is that you likely need to deal with a few other things in your life or relating to your body.

It also means that this book is perfect for you.

Weight Loss is Built on Big Wins

It's very popular these days to talk about or advertise "one little trick" or "one secret found by Harvard researchers."

And it's very tempting to read those articles or buy whatever they're selling, because we'd all love to find the secret solution that we've been missing.

But the problem is that those "little" tricks produce "little" results. Sometimes, somebody will get lucky and get big results, but that's the exception rather than the rule.

This book is not filled with little tricks or secret techniques. Instead, it's filled with tactics and practices that are proven to result in *Big Wins*.

Think of it like this: You could spend the rest of your life buying lottery tickets and trying to hit it big. Or . . . you could learn proven techniques for earning more and then growing your investments.

If you choose to play the lottery, most of your results will actually be very small wins (or nothing at all). A few people will get lucky, but most will lose far more money than they ever win.

On the other hand, learning to earn more and to invest well will almost always result in big wins over time.

Weight loss is no different. You need a clear and proven path to big wins, rather than little tricks. And that's exactly why I've written this book: **to show you a clear path to weight loss (and to greater overall health)**.

There are other good weight loss books out there, but very few that have a complete system (encompassing more than just diet—health, exercise, psychology, and more) for weight loss.

The process in this book has worked amazingly well for thousands of people. But before you jump in, there's one big thing to remember . . .

It's OK to Want to Lose Weight

Wanting to lose weight or just look better does <u>not</u> make you a bad person.

It doesn't really matter why you want to lose weight, whether it's to look more attractive, feel more comfortable with yourself, or to be healthier.

If you want to lose weight, then that's what you want. And that's ok. No matter what the reason, don't beat yourself up about wanting to lose weight, because that will lead to sure failure in the long run.

Most of us are incredibly ashamed that we want to lose weight or to look better. We tell ourselves that we shouldn't care how we look or what other people think.

But that's irrelevant because it doesn't change what you want. And the worst part is, those thoughts and beliefs are holding you back.

If you believe (even subconsciously) that you shouldn't want to lose weight, then your mind will find all sorts of ways to make you fail.

Your brain finds ways to sabotage your weight-loss efforts if—*deep down*—you believe that you shouldn't want to lose weight. You'll have less willpower to resist temptation, you'll find excuses not to eat healthy or exercise, you'll be more stressed, and you won't sleep as well. Your beliefs are *that powerful.*

Most of this book is about practical actions you can take to start losing weight now. However, everything else I show you won't make a difference if you're continually sabotaging yourself.

So What Should You Do?

Chapters 5 and 16 are all about getting in the right state of mind to lose weight.

However, you must start by simply acknowledging if you feel even a little bit guilty about wanting to lose weight.

If you don't acknowledge feeling bad in the first place, then you'll never get over it. Ask yourself questions like:

- Am I afraid to tell people that I'm trying to lose weight?
- Do I have thoughts like "I should just be OK with myself and accept myself the way that I am"?

If you find yourself thinking these things, then just notice it. Simply noticing how you feel will go a very long way toward letting it go.

Even apart from losing weight, you probably shouldn't ever feel bad about wanting anything, because we typically don't control what we want. You don't wake up in the morning and decide what to want or not want. You just want it.

So as you read the rest of this book and start to implement it in your life, just be aware of any "*shoulds*" or "*shouldn'ts*" that you feel along the way—any time that you feel like you ought to do something, rather than wanting to do it to achieve your goal.

Chapter 2

COMMON SENSE AND UNCOMMON RESULTS

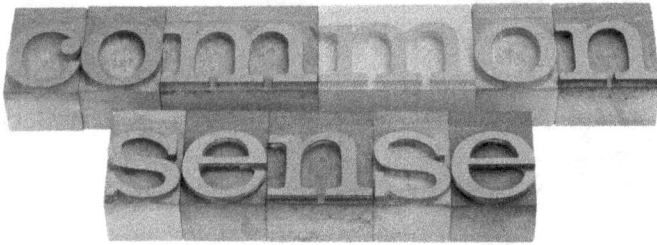

"What is Common Sense is Not Always Common Practice."
—*Stephen Covey*

Y OU DO MANY things that you know you shouldn't do.

- You stay up too late watching a TV show.

- You eat a food that you know will make you feel bad.

- You yell at a family member for something small they do.

It's normal. You're human. But we need to remind ourselves that the problem is not usually *knowing* what to do.

The problem is actually *doing* what you already know you should.

If you want to lose weight, you need to know what really matters for weight loss. You need to know the big wins that will make the biggest difference. And I'll show you all of that.

Before I do, though, remember this . . .

Boring is Beautiful

A lot of what I'm going to tell you isn't new. It's not a secret, and it's not shocking.

If I wanted to get on TV, I would need to come up with very controversial and unknown tactics. That would make me popular and sell more books.

But it won't help you lose weight. What I'm going to tell you is what's absolutely necessary, whether it's boring or not.

Then, I'm going to show you how to implement everything in your life, so that you can actually stick to it.

This chapter is very short. But it's something you and I often need to reminded of. Because . . .

Big, Boring Wins ↦ Big, Exciting Results

Everything worth having takes work behind the scenes. And it's not glamorous work, even if the results are amazing.

People with amazing bodies don't always eat exciting food. People with successful businesses often do very boring work when you aren't looking. And people with great relationships usually work very hard on those relationships.

Luckily, you're serious about losing weight. And because of that, here are some of the results you can expect from the "Run then Rest" system:

1. **Better Health**. As I mentioned in the Introduction, losing weight is an accident of being healthy. It happens automatically when you get all of the 8 Fundamental Principles right. That took me 20 years, but it's something you can do much faster. And as a result, you can expect much better health in every respect: better blood work, more energy, less illness, and more.

2. **Quick Results**. There are 2 big reasons why my system delivers fast results. First of all, you're going to focus on the "Big Wins." These are the things that will make the biggest difference for your body, rather than changes that make very little difference. Second, I'll show you how to quickly reduce bloating and inflammation. So in addition to any weight that you lose, you'll also *look* lighter very quickly.

3. **Stress-Free**. Let's be honest. Most diets are stressful. You feel like you don't get enough food and like you're fighting your body. With the "Run then Rest" system, you only focus on 2-3 things at a time. And if you fall off the wagon, you simply take a very short break and then start one of the phases over again.

4. **Repeatable Results**. Sometimes life happens. You might get sick for a few weeks. Or you'll eat badly on vacation or while traveling for work. When that happens, you can rest easy knowing that you can simply start a new "phase"

and start getting results again. This isn't magic—if you eat junk food for 2 months, you'll probably gain some weight. But the beauty is that if you do, you now have the tools to recover from it.

5. **Automatic Weight Loss**. Again, this isn't magic. But humans aren't designed to worry about how much they eat and exercise every day. It's tiring and drains your willpower. I'm going to show you how to focus on just a few things at a time and build habits into your life that will cause weight loss to happen when you're not even thinking about it.

Listen . . .

I can't promise or guarantee any results. Most people won't read this entire book, and many of the people who do won't put it into action.

But I'm going to make it as simple and easy as possible for you to do this and to set yourself up for amazing results. Weight loss is never easy, or else we wouldn't have so many problems with obesity. It is possible to lose weight and keep it off, though. I'm proof of that, and so are many of the people with whom I've worked.

You can do this, and you can be happier with your body than you've ever been.

Chapter 3

8 TERRIBLE MYTHS ABOUT WEIGHT LOSS

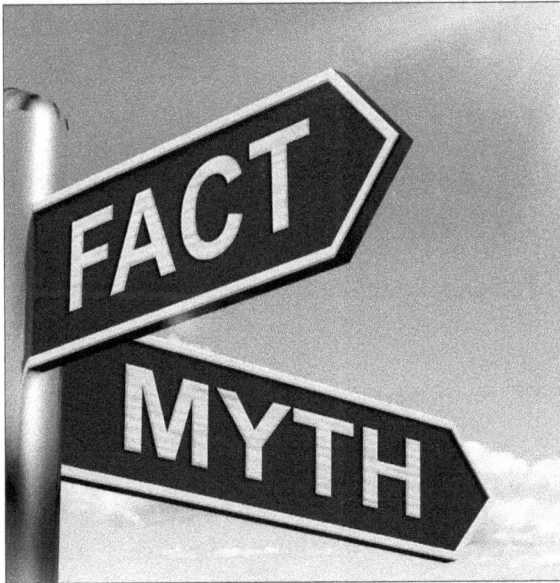

I HATE BAD INFORMATION. But it's gotten much worse lately, especially on the internet. When one person makes up a fake fact, then a million other people start repeating it.

All of a sudden, everybody believes something that was never true to begin with. And it's a big problem, particularly when it comes to weight loss. Not only do people have *bad* information, but they stop really believing that anything will work for them. They become incredibly skeptical.

For example, many people start a diet because they've heard how awesome it is. And yet, they don't actually believe that it will work. Many people I talk to say that they'll "give it a go." Here are a few real quotes from people . . .

> *"I saw it on Facebook, a couple of people I know were doing it. Thought I'd give it a go."*

> *"It worked for her including weight loss and better health so i decided to give it a go as well"*

> *"My girlfriend mentioned it and we decided to give it a go"*

What these people really mean is that they'll "give it a go" for a few days, but if they don't see any quick results, then they'll try something else.

And because of this noncommittal attitude, when things don't work out as quickly as they had hoped, they often fall prey to the many myths that surround diet and give up.

And because they start off with those beliefs, they never give the diet or lifestyle a chance. They do it half-heartedly, and when it gets tough, they give up very quickly.

I don't want that to happen to you. And in order to avoid that, we need to talk about a few myths . . .

Myth #1: Diet Alone is Enough

This is a very popular myth, especially if you eat a Paleo or real-food diet. I think it got started because there was a backlash against exercising for hours everyday to lose weight. Bloggers and authors tried to put the emphasis back on diet rather than exercise.

Generally, that was a good thing. In many ways, what we eat is the most important part of losing weight. But that doesn't mean it's enough. There are many other things that are also necessary for your body to lose weight with ease. Sometimes people can lose weight without everything being in place, but often not.

So if all of your focus right now is on what you're eating or not eating, then it's likely because part of you believes that once you get your diet perfect, you'll lose weight and feel better. I've been there myself. For almost a decade, I kept thinking that if I could just make my diet a little bit better, then everything would fall into place.

I learned the hard way that diet is necessary, but it's not sufficient.

Myth #2: More Exercise is Better

Even though most dieters now believe that "chronic cardio" is the wrong way to lose weight and get healthy, many folks still believe that exercising for hours a day is critically important for weight loss. Often, this takes the form of running, aerobics classes, CrossFit, or similar activities.

Those are all fine things to do. But let's be clear—you don't actually *need* to do loads of exercise. You might do those activities because you enjoy them, because you want to compete in them, or for many other reasons, and that's fine.

In fact, it's possible in some cases that doing too much intense exercise can create the same type of inflammation in your body as a chronic infection—inflammation that generally makes it harder for your body to shed unwanted pounds.

To some degree, if you exercise enough, it will always help you lose weight. For instance, you'll see very few overweight people who cycle hundreds of miles every week. My friend Chris is a professional cyclist who rides a LOT, and he'd have a hard time putting on fat if he tried.

But doing that much exercise is not necessarily the *best* way to lose weight, and it's likely something that you won't be able or willing to keep up. Besides, if you were willing and able to do that much exercise, you probably wouldn't be reading this book right now.

What this means for you depends on how addicted to exercise you are. If you're at the gym every single day, then great—just take a look at how you feel and whether you're getting stronger or whether you feel tired all the time. If it's the latter, then you probably need to cut back just a little.

On the other hand, if you don't exercise at all, then I'll also talk about how some exercise is almost essential. And if you're in between those 2 extremes, then you might not need to change as much.

I'll cover exactly how to approach exercise for weight loss in Chapter 7.

Myth #3: Calories are All that Matters

There are so many myths around calories that I barely know where to begin. In fact, one of the most popular questions I get asked by people who are starting a Paleo diet is how many calories they should eat each day.

Unfortunately, many of these myths come from blogs and books. One of the biggest myths is that calories don't matter at all (which runs against the popular myth that calories are all that matter). Neither of these myths are true.

It definitely matters how much you eat. If you're eating 5,000 calories a day, it's nearly impossible to lose weight.

Still, it also matters where those calories come from. If you eat 2,000 calories per day of cookies, you're going to look different than if you eat 2,000 calories per day of vegetables and seafood. We all know this is true.

The problem is not that calories don't matter—it's that counting calories usually doesn't work.

Fortunately, a *good* diet helps your body automatically regulate calories. And that's an excellent thing, because humans are not very good at voluntarily controlling how much we eat. We're just not wired to keep resisting food when it's available.

In general, I won't talk about calories much at all in this book. It's not because I think they don't matter. Most people just don't have very much success with counting calories. It's not part of the process that I've seen help so many people to lose weight and get healthy.

As I said, it's not because calories don't matter but rather because failure is almost guaranteed if you're constantly trying to limit the amount you eat when you're hungry. It just doesn't work over the long term.

Myth #4: You Shouldn't Eat Fat/Carbs

Like calories, there are more myths than I can count about fat and carbs. Scientifically, every single study shows that when all else is equal, you can lose weight with both low-fat and low-carb diets.

If you're just starting out, then chances are that you're still at least a little bit afraid of fat. And that's understandable, because the media has beaten into us for years that eating fat makes us fat (and also leads to other bad things like high cholesterol, heart disease, etc.). Luckily, none of that is true. Fat is a necessary part of the human diet, and many of the most important vitamins (A, D, E, K) you only get from fat.

Carbs are also not something to be afraid of. I often recommend low-carb diets because they make it easier for many people to control their hunger, cravings, and energy—particularly if you have high blood sugar or low insulin sensitivity. But if you're an athlete who needs short bursts of power, carbs are probably necessary for you to compete at your best.

Lowering or raising your carbs is simply a tool that helps folks lose weight and feel better. It doesn't mean you need to be afraid of carbs. In fact, many people (myself included) look and feel much better when we're eating some carbs.

Myth #5: Genetics

Many members of my own family believe that they're destined to be overweight because of their genetics. It's partially an excuse, but it's also something that they truly believe.

Here's the truth: Genetics plays a role, but *only* a role. Both your genetics and your epigenetics (how your genes express themselves) can make you more or less likely to be overweight or not.

But your genes are NOT determinative. Even though they make something more or less likely, they don't have the final word. You do.

Think of it this way. Your genes might make it more likely that you'll be a really smart scientist, but that will never happen if you never go to school. Or you might be genetically allergic to a food, but it doesn't matter if you never eat that food.

No matter what the rest of your family looks like or what you think you might have inherited, you have full control over your health and your ability to lose weight.

Myth #6: Everything is OK in Moderation

This is one of the myths that annoys me most. Let me give you an example . . .

If you punch yourself in the face just a few times, it probably won't cause any lasting damage. You're doing it in moderation, rather than in excess, right? But why would you do it in the first place?

Eating a piece of cake or drinking a soda is not a "healthy" thing to do, even in moderation. Sleeping for 4 hours per night is not "healthy." There are completely justifiable reasons why you might do those things, just not because moderation is ok.

Remember, you don't have to be perfect to lose weight. If you cheat every once in a while or sleep too little one night, that's not going to destroy all of your progress. But you should consciously choose to do those things because they're fun, necessary, or just worth it. The point is not to beat yourself up.

At the same time, don't justify being unhealthy by acting like it's healthy to do it in moderation.

Myth #7: Willpower

One of the most common things I hear people say is that they don't have the willpower to stick to something. They're just not "strong enough."

Once you believe that, you've already lost the game. Because if you believe you're not going to be able to do it, then your brain is going to find a way to make sure that you can't do it. That's how your subconscious mind works. It makes sure that reality fits what you believe to be true.

The sad part is, getting healthy is not about willpower. If you try to rely solely on willpower to stick to your plans, it's pretty obvious what's going to happen. You're going to fail like you have in the past. Take it from me—I tried to rely on willpower for the first few years I was on a Paleo diet, and I'd regularly fall off the wagon for a month or two at a time.

Getting healthy is all about putting the right systems in place. It's about focusing on the Big Wins, holding yourself accountable, forgiving yourself when you fail, and creating habits that happen without you even thinking about it.

None of this happens in a day, but all of the people who are most successful at losing weight are able to put these types of systems in place. In Chapter 5, I'm going to talk exclusively about your mindset.

The entire chapter will help you build a system that makes sure you don't need to rely on willpower any more.

Myth #8: Certain Foods are Stored as Fat

ALL foods can be stored as fat. PERIOD.

If you eat a spoonful of sugar, and your body already has enough sugar, that sugar will be converted and stored as fat. If you eat a protein shake or bar, some of that protein might be used for muscle repair, but any protein you don't need will be converted and stored as fat. And if you drink a tablespoon of coconut oil, any energy you don't immediately need will be stored as fat.

That's just how your body works. If you couldn't store food as fat, it would be generally useless for your body. You would need to be eating 24 hours a day. Fat in your body is where you get energy from when you haven't just eaten.

So don't worry about whether or not a particular food can be stored as fat. They all can.

Just worry about whether or not a particular food is going to make you more or less healthy—something I'll cover in detail in Chapter 6.

Myth #9: Endless Dieting

Very often, I'll talk to someone who is very disappointed with themselves. Usually, they were really good with their diet and exercise for several weeks or months, and then something caused them to "fall off the wagon."

And so this person will start beating themselves up.

You've probably found yourself in that situation. Either you ran out of willpower (Myth #7 above), or else life just happened (vacation, travel, illness, etc.).

The problem is that these people believe they can diet forever. They cannot and you cannot.

As humans, we've evolved to eat food when it's available. Your ancestors survived famines because of that trait. But for you, it means that you can't diet forever—you're not going to have the willpower or motivation to always resist temptation.

That's why I created the Run then Rest approach, and that's why it works. It allows you to be strict for a while and then relax and allow your body to adjust to being healthier and leaner.

Chapter 4

THE 8 FUNDAMENTAL PRINCIPLES OF EFFECTIVE WEIGHT LOSS

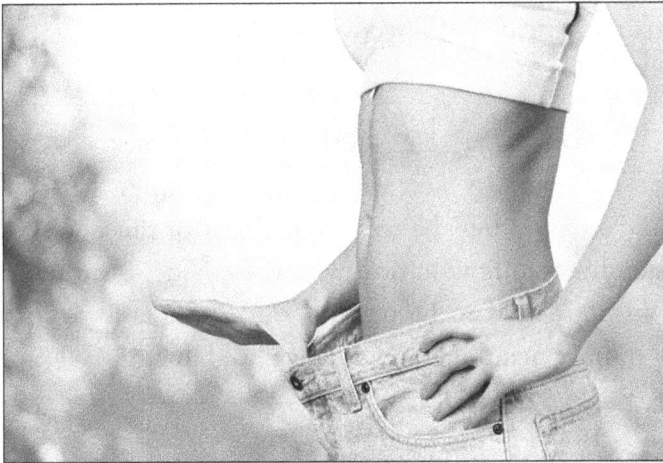

IMAGINE THAT YOU have a car sitting in your garage. Your car has **no tires, no gas**, and **no battery**.

One day, you decide to fix your car, so you have it towed to your local mechanic.

After he inspects your car, he comes over and says "Your car definitely needs new tires, and we can help you with that." You agree, and next thing you know, your car has a new set of tires.

You happily pay the mechanic, hop in, and try to drive off. Only problem is . . . your car still won't go anywhere.

This is a rather silly story, since it's very obvious that your car won't go anywhere without a new battery and some gas.

However, the same thing happens with our bodies. Even if you're eating the best possible diet for your body, there could still be a number of things that are making it very hard for your body to lose weight.

That's why I want to talk first about diet before jumping into the 8 Fundamental Principles of Effective Weight Loss . . .

PLEASE!: Do NOT let yourself be overwhelmed by this chapter. I'm going to mention quite a few things that could be holding you back, but the entire remainder of this book will tell you (step-by-step) how to deal with these issues. And remember that you don't need to be perfect. You might need to focus on several things I mention, but you don't need to be at 100% perfect health.

CLARIFICATION: This chapter covers the basics of what the 8 Fundamentals are, but Chapters 5-12 will show you Big Wins in each area of your life as well as explain many of the fundamentals in more detail. These Big Wins are the changes that will help you achieve the 8 Fundamentals Principles of Effective Weight Loss.

Diet is Just One Aspect of Your Health

Quite often, someone will email me saying that they're trying to lose weight, that they've been eating a real-food or Paleo diet for a long time (at least a couple months), and that they're not seeing any results.

And usually, they'll ask if they're doing something wrong or if the diet just isn't for them.

One thing is for sure—eating real, whole foods that are high in nutrients and low in toxins is the right thing to do for EVERY HUMAN. So unless you're not human, eating real, whole, unprocessed food can't be the wrong thing to do.

But that doesn't mean that a good diet is enough. There's a big difference between <u>good for you</u> and <u>good enough</u>. For instance, rain is good for a flower, but if it only rains one day per year, it's probably not good enough.

Some folks can change what they're eating and almost immediately see big changes to their body. You've probably read success stories online, and you might even know somebody who's had that kind of success. The story often sounds like this . . .

Your friend used to eat a Standard American Diet. They woke up one day and decided to cut out all the processed junk food and eat only real foods like vegetables, meats, fruits, and seafood. As soon as they do, they suddenly have way more energy, they heal illnesses that they've been battling for years, and they lose a LOT of fat.

Many of those stories are very real—I've talked to or emailed thousands of people with amazing results.

However, that's not the reality for everybody (or even most people).

In this chapter, I'm going to show you the **8 Fundamental Principles of Effective Weight Loss** that might be missing from your life and might be sabotaging your efforts at weight loss. These are the fundamentals that you need to get right in order to be healthy and lose weight.

You likely already have some of these fundamental principles in place in your life, but don't worry if they seem like a lot. I'll show you exactly how and when to implement each principle in the other chapters of this book.

Fundamental Principle #1: Automatically Control Hunger

The human body evolved over 2.5 million years. And during 99% of that time, food was scarce and *never* addictive.

Today, most of your food is manufactured in bulk. The goal is to be as addictive as possible for you. It's why the biggest food companies in the world hire food scientists to make food "hyper-palatable."

"Hyper-palatable" doesn't just mean that the food tastes good. After all, steak tastes good, but there's only so much steak you can eat.

Hyper-palatable means that food is addictive. You'll keep eating even when you don't need the food or have eaten enough.

So you now live in a world of plentiful, ultra-addictive food.

That's why Fundamental Principle #1 is to <u>control your hunger without needing to constantly fight it</u>.

Your body and brain haven't evolved to resist addictive food. Your willpower is limited, and your brain wants to eat whenever it feels the need or urge.

This is why counting calories doesn't typically work. You can't keep it up, because your willpower eventually gives out.

The solution is not to build more willpower. The solution is to teach your body to automatically regulate your hunger (like it is built to do).

In fact, several of the other Fundamental Principles will help with this too. Reducing inflammation, for instance, reduces hunger. Balancing your hormones also reduces hunger, because your brain becomes more sensitive to hormones like leptin and ghrelin, which help control hunger.

But there are also other Big Wins you can implement to automatically regulate your hunger. And throughout the rest of this book, I'll show you many of those Big Wins and just how easy they are to implement, so that you're less hungry without even thinking about it.

Summary

Fundamental Principle of Effective Weight Loss #1: Hunger is not something you want to fight because it's a losing battle. Instead, you want to put your body in a position to automatically regulate your hunger so that you're only hungry when you need energy and nutrients, rather than when you get stressed, tired, or see a donut.

Fundamental Principle #2: Minimize Chronic Inflammation

Inflammation is both very good and very bad for your body.

If you sprain your ankle or scrape your knee, then your body will respond by causing your ankle or knee to swell up. That's inflammation, and it's a very good thing.

That type of inflammation makes infection less likely and assists in healing the injury. Plus, that type of inflammation goes away after a few days, once it's done its job.

On the other hand, chronic inflammation in your body is at the root of almost every chronic illness, and it's the main thing that will keep you from losing weight. A few years ago, I interviewed Dr. Dwight Lundell (a surgeon) who has performed <u>thousands</u> of open-heart surgeries.

During our interview, I asked him if there were any common factors he saw among all of his open-heart surgeries, and this was his reply:

"Every one of [my open-heart surgery patients] had the cardinal signs of inflammation. Now those four cardinal signs are redness, swelling, warmth, and pain. Now in places in our bodies we can't feel it, but there was certainly redness and swelling . . . in all 5,000 of those hearts" (that Dr. Lundell performed surgery on).

Inflammation. In every single case.

Fundamental Principle #2 is to <u>reduce and minimize chronic inflammation</u>.

From heart disease to diabetes to autoimmune disorders, inflammation is one of the primary causes. And this is chronic inflammation, which doesn't go away like the inflammation of a cut or bruise.

This type of inflammation is largely invisible, although you may see signs of it in the form of arthritis, dermatitis, or even acne.

When it comes to weight gain/loss, inflammation plays a huge role.

Even if you're eating a near-perfect diet (with no inflammatory grains, sugars, or seed oils), your body could still be subject to chronic inflammation. If that's the case, then weight loss is going to keep being very hard for you.

First of all, *inflammation causes insulin resistance*, which make weight loss incredibly hard and also leads to diabetes. Inflammation does this in two ways: (i) first, by causing your fat cells to release a small protein that directly causes fat cells to become insulin resistant, and (ii) second, by causing your gut to produce lipopolysaccharide (a fat and sugar molecule), which directly leads to insulin resistance in the liver.

If that weren't bad enough, *inflammation also causes leptin resistance*. Leptin is largely responsible for helping to control how much you eat and how much energy you burn, so leptin resistance is a big problem for weight loss. Inflammation causes leptin resistance by causing a portion of your brain to become less sensitive to leptin.

In addition to all of that, chronic inflammation also keeps your body in a fight-or-flight state. When in this state, your body does everything it can to protect the fat that you already have so that it can survive for longer if you don't have food for a while (not a likely scenario today, but your body doesn't know that).

Inflammation also makes you hungry and tired, which means you snack more and move less.

Almost everything bad that happens in your body is either caused by inflammation or at the very least results in inflammation. And most of us are walking around with a lot more inflammation than we know.

Inflammation is caused by bad diets, too little sleep, too much stress, too much exercise, parasites and other pathogens, and a lot of other culprits. Everything in this book is designed to reduce the inflammation in your body.

Almost every chapter remaining in this book will deal either directly or indirectly with inflammation, because it's that important. And almost every Big Win that you'll implement during a Dash will be designed to reduce inflammation, among other things.

But in the meantime, try to start being more aware of how inflammation is affecting you. That way, you'll eventually be more aware of when something has caused you to become inflamed, and you'll be able to easily identify the culprit.

Summary

Fundamental Principle of Effective Weight Loss #2: Inflammation is not only the root cause of most major illness, but also keeps your body from losing weight. Chronic inflammation can be caused by too little sleep, a bad diet, over-exercise, infection, and many other culprits. The entire approach laid out in this book is designed to reduce inflammation.

Fundamental Principle #3: Improve Your Gut Health

A very long time ago, Hippocrates said that all illness begins in the gut.

Then, for about 2,000 years, we pretty much forgot that lesson.

If inflammation is the biggest cause of weight gain (and other health issues), then poor gut health is the biggest cause of inflammation.

Fundamental Principle #3 is to <u>improve and optimize your gut health</u>.

Your gut—including your stomach and intestines—is the barrier between the "outside" world and your bloodstream. In other words, food you've just eaten is still "outside" your body. It's inside your gut, but it hasn't yet been allowed into your bloodstream.

One of the primary problems is that your gut will occasionally allow things into your bloodstream that it shouldn't, such as undigested food, bacteria, and viruses. When that happens, your body reacts by going on high alert and starting to attack those things that made it through by accident. And that results in a lot of inflammation.

Also, your gut is home to trillions of bacteria and other micro-organisms, all of which actually help your body to break down food and fight off infection. However, if these bacteria get out of control, or if too many of them die off, then you run into a lot of problems. You can't break down certain foods, you can't fight off bad bacteria and other micro-organisms, and your immune system (which is somewhat reliant on your gut bacteria) doesn't work as well. And you can guess what that all leads to . . . Inflammation.

The most important thing to remember about your gut is that it keeps bad things out (pathogens, undigested food) and lets good things in (vitamins, minerals). When your gut stops doing these things well, you become deficient in vitamins and minerals, you start developing illnesses, and you become chronically inflamed.

And all of those outcomes make it significantly harder to lose weight. Fortunately, a good diet is a great first step for healing your gut. But it's not always enough—by itself—to undo any damage that's already been done. (And depending on what your diet looks like, you might need to improve that as well.)

Also, when you improve your gut health, you'll see quicker results in terms of appearance and weight loss than with any other fundamental.

Summary

Fundamental Principle of Effective Weight Loss #3: Poor gut health is a huge cause of inflammation, illness, and trouble with weight loss. Improved diet, sleep, and sometimes supplementation can quickly and dramatically improve this area of your life.

Fundamental Principle #4: Stay Hydrated

The most boring principle is also the easiest one to fix . . .

Water.

You might be skeptical that water could help you lose weight. I personally understand that very well, and this was one of the last changes I made in my own life. We all know that water is important, but it's very easy to forget.

But staying hydrated is critically important for your ability to lose weight for a variety of reasons:

- Water helps reduce inflammation.

- Water helps you think better and more clearly (just 1-2% dehydration leads to cognitive decline in studies).

- Water—if you drink it at the right times—helps control hunger.

- Water actually affects how your genes are expressed and how your cells function.

And those are just some of the reasons that modern science has proven that water helps with health, mindset, and weight loss.

You need to know all of this to really understand how important it is to be hydrated on a DAILY basis. In other words, it's not ok to be hydrated some days and then not others. That would be like eating cake and cookies 3 days a week while eating healthy the other 4 days. It doesn't balance out.

So hydration needs to be an all-the-time thing, which means that drinking sufficient water needs to be done on a daily basis.

You might notice that I haven't said how much water you need to drink, and that's because it varies a lot depending on your weight, your activity level, and several other factors. However, I haven't yet met any adults who needed less than 2 liters per day.

> **Summary**
>
> Fundamental Principle of Effective Weight Loss #4: Hydration is essential for your cells, brain, and body to function properly. You must drink enough water every single day.

Fundamental Principle #5: Balance Your Hormones

Your hormones are not directly under your voluntary control. You can't just think in the right way and have your body produce more cortisol or be more sensitive to leptin.

And yet hormones are incredibly important for helping you lose weight and get healthy.

I won't go into too much detail here, but hormones are essentially the messengers of your body. They're usually produced in one part of your body (or a couple places) and then tell other parts of your body what to do. That's an oversimplification, but you get the idea.

For instance, cortisol tells your body to be alert, not to sleep, and to produce or release more sugar. Leptin tells your body to stop eating and use more energy. You've got hundreds of hormones in your body, and they're all important, but certain hormones get messed up more easily than others and stall your weight loss.

One of the biggest ways that your hormones can keep you from losing weight is by making you hungry or tired. I'll show you easy ways to decrease your hunger and increase your energy. And when you do, you'll eat less and move more without even thinking about it.

A good diet will go a long way toward fixing your hormones, but it's not always enough. Other aspects of your lifestyle (sleep, stress, etc.) are also critical. Even beyond lifestyle, though, you may need to do a bit of testing to figure out what's going on with your hormones and how to fix them.

I'll cover all of the Big Wins to get your hormones in order in the following chapters.

Summary

Fundamental Principle of Effective Weight Loss #5: Hormones control much of your health and almost all of your weight loss. They're influenced by food, exercise, sleep, and particularly stress, but you also have the ability to order tests that will allow you to directly address any concerns.

Fundamental Principle #6: Maintain Muscle Mass and Bone Density

Do you remember all those exercise videos during the 80s and 90s, from folks like Richard Simmons and Jane Fonda?

The theory was that if you could just exercise enough, then you'd lose weight and be healthy. Of course, we now know that's not true. You simply **cannot** out-exercise a bad diet or a lack of sleep, for instance.

But that does NOT mean you shouldn't exercise or pay attention to moving your body. In fact, one of the single best indicators of how healthy you are (especially as you get older) is how much "lean tissue" you keep. "Lean tissue" is just another way of saying bone plus muscle.

Lean tissue is incredibly important for losing weight.

Generally, the more muscle and bone your body has, the more calories you will burn, and the less likely you will be to gain or regain fat. However, the bigger issue is that most people who lose weight don't lose just fat. They also lose a lot of muscle and bone.

It's almost impossible not to lose *some* lean tissue while you're losing weight, but you must keep it at a minimum. Every Big Win in this book will help you do that, and by doing so, you'll not only look and feel better, but you'll also be much less likely to regain any weight that you lose.

If you're a woman, don't stress out that you're going to get too muscular. Unless you're eating a LOT, working out a lot, and also have some genetic predisposition, it's simply not going to happen. And even if it does, there's a simple solution—work out a bit less.

In the end, maintaining lean tissue is going to require you to move a little more and periodically do some things that feel physically hard. It doesn't mean that you'll spend hours in the gym (or necessarily go to the gym at all), but it does mean that you'll have to do a little bit of working out.

Summary

Fundamental Principle of Effective Weight Loss #6: Lean tissue is critical for both your overall health and also your ability to lose weight and keep it off. I'll show you the easiest and best ways to build and maintain bone and muscle, but don't underestimate how important this is.

Fundamental Principle #7: Getting the Right Mindset

Your mind is arguably even more important to your weight loss efforts than inflammation or gut health. After all, it's your mind (and mindset) that even allows you to stick to a diet, right?

Health and your mind is really a two-way street.

First of all, **your brain is part of your body, so how you treat your body always affects your brain**.

For instance, if you drink alcohol, it immediately changes the way that your brain thinks and reacts. You probably already believe as much, but the same is true of almost any inflammatory food, from gluten to vegetable oil. All of these foods cause inflammation that stops your brain from functioning properly.

Secondly, **how you think also affects your body**.

To begin with, if you *believe* that you're unhealthy or sick, then you're far more likely to actually be or become sick. And there is a lot of science proving that this is the case, even though we're still not 100% sure how this happens. However, we definitely know some of the ways our brain affects our body and our health.

You have a part of your brain called the Reticular Activating System (RAS). The RAS controls what you focus on, what you notice, and in the end, what you experience. Right now, you could notice a million different things in your world. But you only notice and experience a few of them.

This is a very powerful concept. You don't just interpret what you see or hear differently—you actually see and hear different things.

So what does this mean for your health and weight loss?

Ironically, the *first* step for losing weight is to believe that you're healthy and losing weight—even before you start. Because if you can start to believe that you're getting healthier and losing weight, you will actually cause your body to find ways to do so. It's not magic, but it will seem like it.

Plus, if you can believe that you're losing weight, you'll also be much happier and more motivated. It's a win-win scenario.

And in Chapter 16, I'll give you a powerful technique to start changing your mind so that your body will follow.

If you need more encouragement, also note that the state of your mind—particularly a stressful state—directly induces inflammation in your body and makes it harder for you to lose weight. So we'll be talking a fair amount about stress control and management.

Summary

<u>Fundamental Principle of Effective Weight Loss #7</u>: Getting your mindset right ensures that you'll have weight loss success no matter your circumstances. In Chapter 16, I'll show you the biggest thing you can do TODAY to get this in order.

Fundamental Principle #8: Pathogens & Deficiencies

Speaking of testing, one of the other things that I highly recommend testing for is pathogens and micronutrient deficiencies. And I'll show you exactly how and what to test for in Chapter 11.

This book outlines a proven step-by-step system for losing weight and getting healthy. And I could have left out the sections on lab testing, because I know it's not the most popular thing to talk about. When you buy a book, you likely want a system that you can implement at home immediately and for no extra cost.

I understand all of that.

But I've also seen so many people struggling with weight loss for so long that I know a big part of the solution is to test to figure out what's actually going on in your body (and then to fix it—often with the help of someone who knows exactly how to remove pathogens or resolve deficiencies). So if I'd left out any discussion of testing for pathogens, hormonal imbalances, and vitamin deficiencies, then I wouldn't be giving you the entire solution.

When you get to the steps involving testing, please don't ignore or skip them in the hopes that everything else will work on its own. It might, but again, you're playing the lottery instead of investing in your future.

To give you a quick idea of what you'll be testing for, remember that your gut is already host to trillions of bacteria and other micro-organisms. And remember that it's very good that you have them there.

However, sometimes you'll get certain bacteria, parasites, fungus, or other micro-organisms that get out of control. When this happens, your body has to constantly fight them, and your gut doesn't work the way it should. Your body becomes inflamed, overworked, and starts to use all of its resources to fight off infection.

When you're in that state, weight loss is near impossible and you'll start developing other health issues. You'll also start developing vitamin and mineral deficiencies, because your body is using those micronutrients as part of the fight.

It's tempting to think that a perfect diet and lifestyle will cure all of these things—and it might. But it usually doesn't. First of all, none of us live a perfect lifestyle, and secondly, even if we did, it'd take decades to heal some of these issues.

I don't know about you, but I'm not willing to wait that long to get healthy or to lose weight.

Summary

Fundamental Principle of Effective Weight Loss #8: Pathogens and Micronutrient Deficiencies are the most overlooked health concerns that also prevent weight loss. A great diet and a little bit of supplementation can potentially solve these problems. But as I'll discuss, you might also consider running some lab tests.

Extra Note: Medications and Illnesses

Two things are true about illnesses and diseases:

1. Illnesses often make it very tough to lose weight.

2. Most illness can be fully healed, so long as you solve the root issues that were initially causing the illness.

So that's a bit of good news and bad news for you. If you have any sort of illness, it *may* be one of the reasons you're having trouble losing weight. (Although that's not necessarily true.) But on the upside, you can likely heal your body and your illness.

Hardly anybody talks about this, but medications can also make it incredibly hard to get certain aspects of your health under control, including weight loss. This is not true of all medications, and it certainly doesn't mean you should stop taking your medication without first consulting your doctor.

However, you need to learn about the side-effects of whatever medication you're taking. Ask your doctor, but also do your own research and read about side effects that other people are experiencing. Read at least 20-30 different websites—particularly a few forums where people are posting their own experiences.

If you have an illness or are on a medication that you think might be keeping you from losing weight, then please don't get discouraged. Even if it makes it harder for you, it doesn't mean that you should give up. First of all, getting healthier will likely help heal your body, and secondly, nothing is set in stone. Although you might have it harder in some ways, you definitely have it easier in others. Perhaps you have more time, more access to the outdoors, you're a better cook, or something else. It all evens out.

I'm mentioning this because it's *real* and it's something you'll want to deal with regardless of your weight loss goals. However, **I do NOT cover treating illnesses at any point in this book (or anywhere else)**. If you have an illness, do everything you can to get healthy in general, but also consult a doctor or other medical professional.

And I'm not saying that only to protect myself legally. Our modern medical system—although it's not perfect—is excellent, and you shouldn't neglect getting medical treatment for any actual illness. Also, I don't address illnesses or medication because there are far too many medications to talk about all of them.

Summary

Illnesses and Medications are not covered in this book but might make it harder for you to lose weight. Please don't stop any medication without consulting your doctor. Talk to your doctor or other health professional to get these issues under control, but please also take some of it into your own hands—for example by doing more research or using a stricter diet (like GAPS or the Autoimmune Protocol diet) if it makes sense for you.

Putting it All Together

The 8 Fundamental Principles I've laid out in this chapter are all necessary in one way or another for your overall health and ability to lose weight.

With the exception of illnesses, Part 3 will address various areas of life where you can get Big Wins and move the needle for each of these

Fundamental Principles. For now, just understand that there's more to weight loss than simply eating the right foods or hitting the gym often enough. If those were the only pieces of that puzzle that you were missing, then that would make all the difference.

But for the vast majority of people with whom I talk and interact, it's not just one piece that's missing. It's multiple ones.

PART II

THE BIG WINS FOR WEIGHT LOSS

A Few Very Important Notes . . .

The first 4 chapters showed you both the 8 fundamental principles of effective weight loss and what doesn't work to lose weight. That's important, but you care most about what *does* work for weight loss.

In Part 2, I'm going to show you exactly <u>what works</u> and <u>why</u>.

But before you dive in, here are a few ***very important notes***:

1. ***8 Fundamental Principles of Effective Weight Loss.*** Chapter 4 covered the 8 Fundamental Principles necessary to start accidentally losing weight. Those principles are the basis for everything else in this book.

2. ***"Big Wins."*** In chapters 5-12, I'll show you the "Big Wins." The Big Wins are <u>not</u> the same as the Fundamental Principles. The Big Wins are the best and easiest ways to <u>achieve the 8 Fundamental Principles</u>.

3. ***"Small Wins."*** In chapters 5-12, I'll also show you some "Small Wins" for weight loss. Some of these things will surprise you, but I'm ***not*** saying that these things don't matter or that they're not good. All I'm saying is that they're not *as important* as the Big Wins.

Part 2 contains a lot of information. If you want to skip it, then that's fine. I think you'll be better off knowing this stuff, but you could follow the system as outlined in Part 3 without knowing very much.

Chapter 5

YOUR MINDSET & BIG WINS

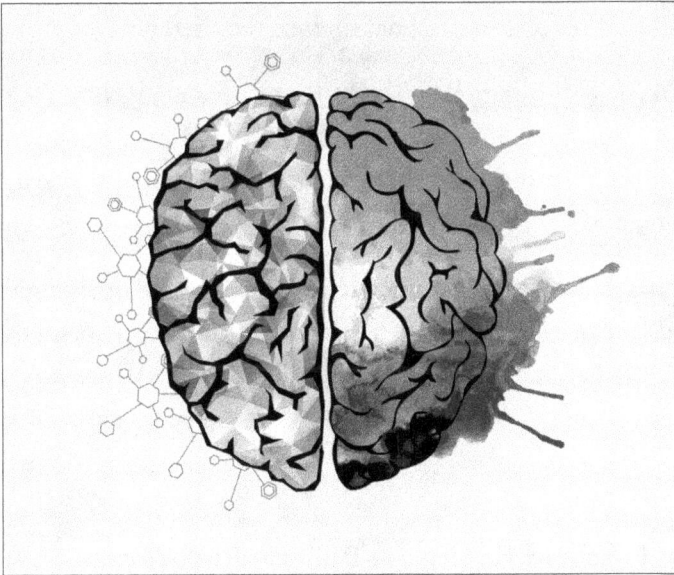

IN THE SUMMER of 2004, Ramit Sethi graduated college at Stanford. By that time, he was already fascinated with both behavior change and personal finance and had already started a website that was growing in popularity.

The whole time, Ramit kept reading and listening to all the advice being given by financial "experts" and "gurus." Experts would tell people to save more money, to buy fewer lattes, and to spend less on shopping.

But no matter how much he tried to educate people, they would always get the same result. **People just weren't following his advice, even if they knew they should.**

In 2009, Ramit wrote and published his first book. Instead of continuing to give the same failed advice, Ramit told people to forget everything they'd been told about personal finance. He told them it wasn't their fault and that success in personal finance required a new approach.

His book, I Will Teach You To Be Rich, became a New York Times Bestseller. But more importantly, Ramit helped tens of thousands of people *successfully* transform their financial lives so that they earn more, save more, and have more time and freedom.

His approach, however, is somewhat surprising. He doesn't give stock tips, and he doesn't care about the small amounts you spend eating or shopping. What he cares about is what he calls **Big Wins.**

And as it turns out . . .

Weight Loss and Health are Built on Big Wins

Big Wins are actions that result in disproportionate gains. In other words, instead of taking a lot of small actions that eventually lead to a result, you take a few bigger actions that get those same results faster and more easily. When you take action on Big Wins, you don't need to worry about the small stuff.

For personal finance, Ramit has a list of Big Wins that includes negotiating a raise, landing a dream job, earning money on the side, and negotiating your rent.

Ramit's approach has changed lives because nobody has the willpower to continually focus on all the small things. But if you can get the Big Wins, then everything else falls into place. After all, if you negotiate a $20,000 raise, you don't really need to worry about how many lattes you drink per day.

Just like personal finance, you can't possibly do everything perfectly when it comes to your diet, exercise, sleep, stress, and the rest of your health.

Your willpower is limited. So if you're trying to (i) exercise an hour per day, (ii) remember to take 30 supplements, (iii) eat perfectly, and (iv) do a hundred other things, then you'll never make it. You don't have the willpower to sustain it.

However, if you can get a few Big Wins in weight loss, then all the small stuff won't matter very much. Everything will start falling into place, and you won't need to rely on willpower continually to make sure that you're doing the little things.

The brilliance of this approach is that once you get a few things right, they benefit you for the rest of your life. It's like having a million dollars in the bank so that you no longer need to worry if your car breaks down or you get a big medical bill.

In terms of health, it means that you don't have to worry about *occasionally* eating badly, missing a workout, or getting too little sleep. You won't beat yourself up for not being perfect, because you'll have systems in your life that allow you to weather any small storm.

Ramit observed the big wins by watching and talking to thousands of people who were trying to change their financial situation. For weight loss, you can learn from the thousands of people I've seen improve their health and lose weight.

That's why this entire section of the book is devoted to Big Wins in various areas of your life (diet, exercise, sleep, etc.)—so that you can do as little as possible to lose weight as quickly as possible. These are the actions that will most quickly and easily allow you to achieve the 8 Fundamental Principles of Chapter 4.

And I'm going to show you 2 Big Wins for your mindset in this chapter. But first . . .

Don't Assume That You're Motivated Enough

Right now, you might feel like you don't need to think about your mindset. You feel the pain of being overweight, and you believe that you have enough motivation to do whatever is necessary to lose weight.

The problem is that your motivation is not going to stay that high. And you know it's true, because you've been here before. You've been excited or serious about losing weight at other times in your life, and for a variety of reasons, you weren't able to follow through.

Part of the reason is because you didn't have the right system in place, and this book will help with that. But part of the reason is also because motivation always goes away at least a little bit.

It's All About Automation, NOT Willpower

The human brain has evolved to have a limited amount of willpower, and your brain is no exception.

It's the reason that most people don't save as much money as they'd like, because when it comes to actually moving the money to a savings or investment account, they can't summon the willpower or motivation to overcome their desire to spend it.

You've probably had the same experience with your health. You want to stick to a diet, but you just can't resist a piece of cake at the party or donuts at the office. Or you want to go to the gym, but you just can't motivate yourself when it's time to go.

And even if you're super-motivated, there will come a time when you're tired, sick, or unhappy, and you won't have much willpower left to stick to the plan.

However, you can absolutely set up systems that keep you from having to use willpower in the first place or that provide you with enough motivation that willpower won't be a concern. For instance, one of the most powerful solutions for saving money is to have the money move <u>automatically</u> from your bank account to your savings account each month. It really works.

Automation is just as important for weight loss and health, but it's also a bit tougher. Fortunately, the Big Wins I'll show in this chapter will help you do exactly that (build automatic systems).

2 Words of Caution

Before you dive into the Big Wins, remember 2 things:

1. **This takes time**. Very rarely do people make dramatic and lasting changes overnight. Instead, we typically go back to our old patterns pretty quickly.

For long-lasting results in your mindset, your health, and weight loss, you need to approach everything with a long-term view. Get excited and make some immediate changes, but also understand that not everything will work perfectly all the time.

This is the entire reason that I developed the Run then Rest approach. You need times when you're strict and building healthy habits, but you also need times when you can take it easy and allow your body to adjust to being thinner.

2. **Mastering the basics is key**. Some of the Big Wins are very basic. You might already be doing some of them in whole or in part.

But the true key to success is to really master the basics and make them second nature. It's the reason that professional athletes practice basic skills every single day, and it's the reason that musicians still practice scales.

Even if you think you are already doing something, really examine your life and ask yourself how you might be able to do it better.

Big Win #1: Get Clear on Your Pain

In order to get and stay motivated, you MUST get clear on the pleasure and pain that will result from doing or not doing what you want to do.

Anything we do in life, we do it either because it brings us enough pleasure or because not doing it will bring us enough pain. Most people go to work because they imagine the pain of not having a job would be greater than going to work. And most people watch TV because they imagine the pleasure of watching will be greater than anything else they want to do at that moment.

You want to lose weight, or else you probably wouldn't be reading this book. And on some level, you know why you want to lose weight, whether it's to look better, feel better, get healthy, or anything else.

But if you want to stay motivated when times are toughest, then your pain and pleasure need to be incredibly deep and visceral. For instance, if someone pinched you every time you were about to eat a donut, then the impending pain would be immediate and visceral.

Fortunately, you don't need anyone to do that. You can actually accomplish that same trick inside of your mind.

In Chapter 16, I've included a simple mental/writing exercise that takes just 30–45 minutes to do. It's so important that I've made it the one thing you need to do IMMEDIATELY. If you want to skip to that exercise now and complete it, please do. Or, you can finish reading the rest of this book and complete it at that time.

But please complete the exercise before you start implementing any of the other Big Wins in the book or the Run then Rest System.

And if you feel like you're losing motivation or willpower at any point, then I encourage you to sit down and do the exercise from Chapter 16 again.

Big Win #2: Hold Yourself Accountable

Of all the things that we hate doing, holding ourselves accountable is near the top of that list. And underneath it all, the primary reason you don't want to hold yourself accountable is because you think you might fail.

For instance, why haven't you told everybody how much weight you're going to lose in the next 12 months? If you haven't, it's because you're scared that you might not do what you say and you might look silly and disappoint your friends or family.

The problem is, if you think you might fail, then your brain will look for ways for you to fail. It will sabotage your diet, lifestyle, and everything else. That's how your subconscious mind works. It looks for ways to match your reality with whatever it believes.

The other reason that you don't make yourself accountable is because you haven't linked enough pain to failing. If you do the pain/pleasure exercises in Chapter 16, the whole point is to make failing so painful that you can't possibly imagine a different outcome. And if you couldn't imagine a different outcome other than success, you wouldn't be scared to hold yourself accountable.

So if you *truly* want to succeed at losing weight, you *must* find a way to hold yourself accountable. Here are 3 ways that I suggest, and you could use any or all of them together:

1. Tell Everybody You Know Your Goal. You don't need to annoy people by telling them constantly, but make it as public as possible. When appropriate, tell your friends, colleagues, and family that you're going to lose __ pounds by _____ date.

What you don't yet realize is that most of these people really want to see you succeed, and telling them will allow them to help you and to cheer you on. In addition, it will make you much less likely to give up when things get hard, because everybody you know will be expecting you to follow through.

And perhaps most importantly, it will start to create a new identity for you. I won't go into the science too much here, but identifying yourself as someone who is willing to do whatever it takes to lose weight will actually train your brain to ignore obstacles and just keep going.

2. Have an Accountability Buddy. If you know someone who is also trying to lose weight or just get healthy, then ask them if they'd like to be your accountability buddy (or however you'd like to phrase it). The point is to talk to each other frequently—at least once a week, but more is better. Check in and see what's going well and what isn't.

Pick somebody that you know, trust, and don't want to let down. But also pick somebody who will be honest with you if you start making excuses or if you slip up too often.

3. Give Money to a Cause You Hate. One of the most motivating ways to follow through is to give a friend some money to hold in case you don't follow through with your plans. You tell them that if you don't succeed (or perhaps if you just don't stick to your plan), that they should donate the money to a cause/charity that you dislike (pick it in advance).

Very few people take this option, because they associate a lot of pain with giving $100 or $1,000 to an organization that they dislike. But that's the point. You want to create extra pain on the side of not acting so that you don't give yourself any way out.

I understand that this seems hard. I always have a lot of resistance to making myself actually accountable. I've avoided it most of my life.

But in those instances where I actually do make myself accountable, I definitely get the results I'm looking for.

And even though so many people criticize programs like weight-watchers, it actually works for a lot of people, and the primary reason it does is because of the accountability that they incorporate into the program.

So ignore your fear, believe in your imminent success, bite the bullet, and just do it.

Small Win: Learn to Forgive Yourself. There is no shortcut for this suggestion that I've ever found for myself or anyone else. But you need to accept now that you're not going to be perfect. Nobody is.

You'll slip up, you'll regress, and you won't always do things the right way. That's OK.

Hopefully you've set up some accountability to make sure that you stay on track even after you slip up. But either way, you need to forgive yourself for not being perfect.

Most of the practices I describe are designed to help you avoid slipping up or giving up, but when you do, you need to gently remind yourself that it's all part of the plan, and you can easily get right back on track without missing a step.

Small Win: These are Life Improvements, Not Temporary Fixes. Remember, losing weight is an accident of living a healthy life. You look great as a side effect of being healthy.

And you aren't healthy by just doing something for a month or a year. You live a healthy life for the rest of your life. If you're just starting out, then that probably sounds daunting, and your mind might be racing with thoughts of giving up cookies and cakes forever.

But that's not the point. First of all, you'll want junk food much less as time goes by. And also, a healthy lifestyle doesn't mean never indulging. Regardless of all that, though, you want to dramatically improve the quality of your life.

You want to look better, feel better, have more energy, and be proud of how you take care of yourself. Those are not feelings that you want to have for only a few months or a year. Those are feelings that you want to last for the rest of your life.

Plus, if you plan on any of these changes being temporary, then you're planning on failure, because you already know what happens when you eat and live the way that you have in the past. You get the same results.

So plan on making permanent changes to your life, but more importantly, plan on seeing permanent improvements to your life.

Small Win: Keep a Journal for a While. You probably don't know this, but in some of the biggest health studies ever done, keeping a food journal is one of the factors that plays the biggest role in whether someone is able to lose weight and maintain weight loss.

In other words, just by recording what you eat every day, you dramatically increase your chances of losing weight and keeping it off.

Keeping a Food Journal is super-easy, and you don't need to do it forever, just for at least 7 consecutive days, 2-3 times a year. Simply record everything that you eat that day. You don't need to record calories or anything like that, but you do need to be completely honest in your food journal about what you ate.

In addition to what you eat, I also highly encourage you to rate how you felt that day on a scale of 1-10. The reason this helps is because it starts showing your brain how certain foods and behaviors affect your body. That way, your brain makes the connections much more quickly, and you start *wanting* to do things that make you feel and look better.

Your Mindset is Critical

Most diet and weight loss books talk a little bit about your mindset, but they don't have a practical system in place for addressing it.

I've adopted these techniques from what I've seen work for many other people and for myself, so I can't take any credit for them, but I wouldn't want to anyway. These are tools that we all have available to us, and we often don't make use of them.

It's tempting to jump right into the diet and lifestyle sections because we believe that those will make the biggest difference. But they don't. Time and again, the people who succeed are those people who have the 3 Mindset Keys in place.

Like everyone else, people who successfully lose weight run into tough times and temptation. But because they feel the pain of failure, because they've automated parts of their health, and because they hold themselves accountable, they're able to get through it all.

Many folks experience brief success by going on a diet or exercising a lot, but it's the ability to build a healthy life that defines long-term success, and you won't get there if your head isn't in the right place.

So if you ever find yourself slipping, please come back to this chapter. These concepts aren't novel or secret, but they're the basic building blocks of any healthy life.

Chapter 6

FOOD & DIET

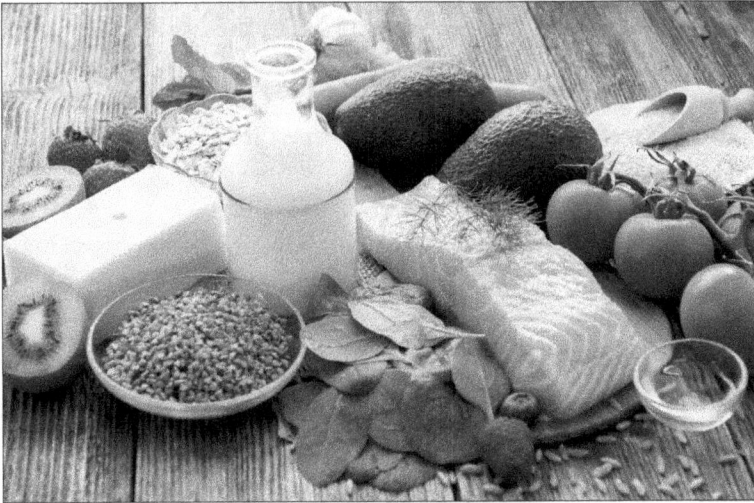

IN 2005, NOVAK Djokovic was 18 years old and playing in one of his first major tennis tournaments. At the time, he was playing the #8 player in the world and was a huge underdog.

Surprisingly, though, Djokovic started off well and won the first set. He looked like he was in control of the match and might pull off a big upset.

However, less than an hour later, Djokovic resigned, saying that he was unable to breathe properly and had lost all of his energy.

Three months later, Djokovic collapsed while playing a match, again being unable to breath and feeling like his body was completely drained.

Djokovic had been experiencing these types of symptoms since he started playing tennis at 6 years old. So Djokovic trained as hard as possible to get in the best shape he could. He ran and biked every single day, changed coaches and training programs, had nasal surgery to improve his breathing, and even moved to the Middle East in order to train in more extreme conditions.

And to a degree, it all paid off. He became the #3 tennis player in the world and won a lot of tournaments.

However, even in 2010, he was still being forced to resign from matches because his body just couldn't keep up.

Luckily for Djokovic, a Serbian nutritionist saw him collapse in one of his tournaments and contacted him with an offer to help. Djokovic agreed to meet, and the nutritionist had him perform a simple test. He had Djokovic hold his right arm straight out to the side. The nutritionist then told Djokovic to try to hold his arm in place while the nutritionist pushed down on the arm. As you might expect for a professional athlete, Djokovic was able to resist a fair amount of pressure.

The nutritionist then held a piece of bread against Djokovic's stomach (touching the skin), and they tried the same exercise. This time, Djokovic was barely able to resist even slight pressure downward on his outstretched arm.

While it's not the most accurate or precise measure of intolerance, it was an easy first sign that Djokovic's body wasn't responding well to wheat at all.

After a few more rigorous lab tests, the nutritionist convinced Djokovic to give up—for 14 days—all wheat and dairy and to cut back on a few other foods. If you're already Paleo or at least gluten free, then you can imagine what happened. Djokovic felt better than ever, started losing weight, gained muscle, and had more energy.

And he never looked back. Just a little over a year after collapsing on court, Djokovic won the biggest tennis tournament in the world and became the #1 ranked player. In fact, that year was one of the best performances EVER, by any player.

One Big Win in Your Diet Can Make a Huge Difference

If you're already eating an amazing diet, then I'm probably preaching to the choir. But no matter where you are, I encourage you to try to make your diet even better.

For Djokovic, wheat and dairy were preventing him from becoming the world's best tennis player. And it took only 2 changes to completely turn around his career and life.

In Chapters 1 and 3, you learned why it might not be enough to just get your diet right. However, weight loss is almost impossible if you don't have your diet dialed in.

In this chapter, I'll show you the **3 Big Wins for Diet**. These Big Wins will *heal* your body and *automatically* help control your appetite, because remember, losing weight is a byproduct of having a healthy body.

> **Side Note**: As with all Big Wins, DO NOT try to do everything at once. Just one of these Big Wins (such as Eliminating Inflammatory Foods) is enough for a single Dash. As a reminder, Part 3 contains a quick-start Guide for the Dashes that I've found most beneficial for weight loss and health.

I'll start by showing you the 3 Big Wins of Diet, because if you're not getting these 3 Big Wins right, then it doesn't make sense to focus on anything else. Definitely implement these 3 Big Wins through the Run then Rest method, because otherwise, you'll get only temporary results. I've seen countless people implement these Big Wins only to later fail because they didn't have a system in place for making sure that these changes stick.

My wife and I have written a lot about the science behind why certain foods make you more or less healthy and more or less likely to lose weight. (You can find most of that information at PaleoMagazine.com.) However, this chapter will not address much of the science, because I want to focus solely on what works.

You might be doing some (or all) of the things outlined in this chapter. If that's the case, then great—focus on other Big Wins.

Just two quick notes before we jump in . . .

Quick Note #1: You Are Not a Unique Snowflake

Well, I'm sure you are in some ways. You're beautiful, talented, and awesome in so many ways.

But when it comes to diet and nutrition, you're mostly the same as everybody else. Nothing I'm going to tell you in this chapter doesn't apply to you—no matter how much you wish it didn't. We'd all love to think that we can eat donuts, pizza, and ice cream without these foods affecting our bodies.

It is NOT the case for you or for anybody else. You might have friends or relatives who eat terribly and yet stay skinny and live a long time. We all know those people in our lives.

The fact of the matter is that those people *could* be much healthier. They could have more energy, they could have more bone and muscle, and they could have a lower risk of disease. Sure, they've gotten a bit lucky that their body is better able to handle the stress and inflammation. But that doesn't mean that it's not affecting them at all.

You might get fat or sick more easily than other people. It's not fair. But it's the way it is.

However, your body will also respond that much better to the Big Wins I'll show you in this chapter. So have faith—you're on the cusp of seeing great results.

Quick Note #2: Inflammation, Energy, and Nutrients

Without getting too deeply into the science, eating food basically does one of two things to your body:

1. Food can provide your body with **nutrients** and **energy**.
2. Food can cause **inflammation** in your body.

Food can do either of these, both of these at the same time, or some combination of the two. But this is a good place to start when you're thinking about food.

Some foods—like alcohol—create a lot of inflammation and supply pretty much zero nutrients. Other foods—such as most vegetables and meats—supply a lot of nutrients and create very little inflammation. Dairy is an example of a food that often does both at once.

Nutrients include everything from protein and fat to vitamins and minerals like A, C, D, K, Magnesium, Zinc, etc.

Inflammation is part of your body's immune response, and it creates all sorts of effects like swelling, redness, pain, or even arterial plaque and cancer growth. In other words, inflammation can be both good and very bad. Chapter 4 covered inflammation to some degree.

Eating one inflammatory food usually won't cause very many noticeable effects. But when you keep doing it over and over again, the effects add up. The result will often be sudden (a heart attack, a new allergy, or another illness), but the cause was built up over many years.

You don't need to understand exactly how inflammation works in your body. However, you do need to understand that it's a cumulative effect. The more inflammatory foods you eat, the worse the results will be over time, and the harder it will be for you to lose weight.

With that, let's jump into Big Win #1 . . .

Big Win #1: Eliminate Highly Inflammatory Foods

For many years, real-food, gluten-free, Paleo, whole-food, and other similar diets have been getting more and more popular.

This is no accident.

The primary way that all these diets work is by removing one or more inflammatory foods. There are other benefits, but that's the biggest win that these diets provide.

And when you remove inflammatory foods from your diet, your body just works better. You have more energy, you get less sick, and you lose weight more easily.

In particular, this Big Win helps you achieve the following Fundamental Principles:

1. Automatically controlling hunger, because inflammatory foods directly and indirectly increase hunger signals.

2. Reducing inflammation.

3. Improving Gut Health, since inflammatory foods often feed the wrong types of gut microbes.

4. Balancing your hormones, because inflammatory foods cause various hormonal responses to deal with the inflammation.

5. Mindset, since inflammation directly affects both your mood and your attitude.

6. Pathologies—eliminating inflammatory foods won't always eliminate pathogens will make it tougher for them to thrive.

For this Big Win, there are 4 foods that are both very common and very inflammatory. But before I tell you what these foods are, you're going to have one big question . . .

"Do I need to stop eating these foods forever?"

The answer is *Yes, But* . . .

You will always need to limit the amount of inflammatory foods you eat, but that doesn't mean you need to forever be without pizza and wine. There are 2 reasons for this:

1. First, if your normal dinner is pizza, cookies and two beers, then you're going to feel bad and look worse. In other words, I can help you lose weight for the next 60 days or even the next year. But if you eventually go back to eating a lot of inflammatory foods, it's going to have an effect. And you already know what that effect will be.

2. Secondly, remember that inflammation is cumulative—it adds up. So if you're only occasionally eating inflammatory foods, then it won't cause as many problems. However, in order to lose weight, you'll need to be very strict during your Dashes.

In other words, don't be worried that you'll never be able to eat pizza again. I've had pizza this year. I didn't feel great after eating it, but I didn't regain all of the weight I've lost either.

So which 4 foods do you need to eliminate for this Big Win?

-   **Food #1: Processed Sugar.**
-   **Food #2: Gluten.**
-   **Food #3: Dairy.**
-   **Food #4: Alcohol.**

These are not the only inflammatory foods. But these are the biggest ones that cause the most problems.

Here's an explanation for each . . .

Processed Sugar

If anyone asks me where to start for weight loss, I almost always suggest removing processed sugar. There are 2 reasons that processed sugar is the first thing I suggest removing, particularly when it comes to weight loss:

1. **Processed Sugar has a huge effect on your brain**. The biggest benefit to giving up processed sugar is that it allows your brain to function more properly. Processed sugar (especially when chronically consumed) reduces the activity in your brain's anorexigenic oxytocin system, which is largely responsible for keeping you full. In addition, excess processed sugar also reduces production of brain-derived neurotropic factor, which leads to insulin resistance.

Those effects of processed sugar (along with a few others) mean that your brain not only doesn't function properly (you don't learn or remember as well), but you also get hungrier and crave more and more sugar.

2. **Processed Sugar has a huge effect on your hormones**. For a variety of reasons, including its effect on your gut bacteria and a tendency to promote insulin resistance, processed sugar can have a very detrimental impact on your hormones. I won't go into much detail on this point, but generally, that detrimental impact leads to lower energy, greater hunger, and greater inflammation.

Together, these 2 effects mean that giving up processed sugar will generally boost your mood and energy and decrease your appetite and cravings. So starting with this step makes everything else easier.

Processed sugar is any sugar that's not naturally occurring in a food. That does not include fruits or things like sweet potatoes, which naturally have sugar in them.

What's the difference?

The difference is that foods that naturally contain sugar have 3 advantages:

1. They almost always have a lot of fiber or water, which make you full and keep you from eating too much sugar.

2. They usually contain most of the nutrients (such as B vitamins) that your body needs in order to properly process sugar.

3. Foods that naturally contain sugar almost never contain very much fat, which automatically keeps you from overeating. (One of the primary reasons we eat too much is because we've started making foods addictive—literally— by combing sugar, fat, and salt in the same food. This pretty much never occurs in any whole food.)

Remember that processed sugar is one of the easiest things to let creep back into your diet, especially if you're eating out or if you start making or buying "healthy" snacks, which often just use "healthy" forms of processed sugar like agave, honey, or coconut sugar. While these forms are marginally better, if you want to lose weight, you're best off still avoiding them.

Here are the many forms of processed sugar to avoid (on any ingredient panel):

- Table sugar;
- Corn syrup;
- Coconut sugar;
- Honey;

- Agave;
- Fructose;
- Sucrose;
- Glucose;
- Beet sugar;
- Rice syrup;
- Brown sugar;
- Cane syrup;
- Caramel;
- Carob syrup;
- Date sugar;
- Galactose;
- Fruit juice concentrate;
- Maltodextrin;
- Maltose;
- Molasses;
- Maple syrup;
- Almost anything with "syrup" in the name.

In the long run, it can be OK to occasionally have a little bit of processed sugar, but if you're serious about losing weight, it's something that you'll want to eliminate completely for a Dash.

Gluten

Hopefully, you're already avoiding gluten. If not, then perhaps Djokovic's story at the beginning of this chapter was enough to convince you.

Depending on how sensitive you are, eliminating gluten may well be the most beneficial change you make in the long run.

When I say to eliminate gluten, I really mean to eliminate all gluten-containing grains (wheat, barley, rye, etc.) and their byproducts (flour, bread, pasta, etc.), because those grains also contain other inflammatory molecules like wheat-germ agglutinin.

For weight loss, eliminating gluten completely (100%) is almost always a necessary step. First of all, it's likely causing some level of inflammation in your body, and we already discussed in Chapter 2 how inflammation will prevent you from losing weight. In addition, like processed sugar, gluten also tends to increase your appetite and make you eat more.

Remember, we're not trying to voluntarily limit the amount we eat. In fact, I usually encourage folks to eat more, which I'll talk about toward the end of this chapter. But when you're eating a great diet (without gluten-containing grains), your body will automatically eat only what it needs and not amounts that will keep you from losing weight.

If you want to know more about the science behind why gluten causes so many problems in your body, I highly suggest starting with this article from Chris Kresser: http://chriskresser.com/50-shades-of-gluten-intolerance.

Otherwise, just try it for a Dash. I've yet to meet anybody who felt worse by removing gluten from their diet, and I'd estimate that upwards of 90% of people who try it feel substantially better. (Ironically, I probably have very little gluten sensitivity myself, and yet it's still something I avoid almost always.)

Dairy

In theory, dairy is highly nutritious. It's got lots of healthy micronutrients, fats, and proteins. And humans have been drinking milk and eating dairy for much longer than we've been eating grains.

But in practice, dairy is a huge problem for a vast number of people, for a couple of reasons. First of all, most modern dairy is pasteurized, which kills all the bacteria and destroys all the enzymes that would help our bodies break down and use dairy. More importantly, though, if your body isn't in ideal condition to begin with, then dairy often exacerbates any problems you already have.

And this has nothing to do with lactose intolerance. It's primarily the casein protein in dairy that causes our bodies to react in an inflammatory way. Once you get healthy and lose all the weight you want to lose, it's entirely possible that you'll be able to tolerate dairy (especially raw and fermented dairy). But until you get there, dairy causes many of the same problems as gluten.

Like gluten, if you don't believe that dairy is causing you any trouble losing weight or with other health issues, then my response is the same. Just try it. For the next 60 days, get rid of all dairy in your life, and see how you feel. Then, after 60 days, try drinking some milk. See if you feel any fatigue or joint stiffness or sinus congestion (all common signs that dairy is causing inflammation in your body).

Alcohol

It's amazing how many people would rather give up every bit of food they eat than to stop drinking alcohol. And when I was younger and partying all the time in New York City, I couldn't have imagined giving up alcohol either. I understand that alcohol is very much a part of many social interactions, and that avoiding it altogether can seem not only hard to do, but also alienating.

So I'm not going to sugar-coat it and make it sound easy. But if you're serious about losing weight and getting healthy, alcohol has no part in that. Ignore all the news about how alcohol may make you healthier in some way or another—it all ignores your main goal (to lose weight).

Alcohol is toxic to your body in very small amounts. What that means is that your body has to put it through a detoxification pathway that uses up valuable vitamins and minerals and that also causes inflammation. If that isn't enough, alcohol is full of junk calories and it generally leads to poor sleep and bad eating choices. You don't need to give up alcohol forever. Just until you lose the weight you want to lose, at which point you might not actually want to add it back.

Summary

Eliminate Highly Inflammatory Foods: This is probably the biggest of the Big Wins I'll give you in this book. If you're on a real-food or Paleo diet, you might already be removing these foods. If not, commit to a 60-day Dash removing these 4 highly inflammatory foods: processed sugar, gluten, dairy, and alcohol.

Big Win #2: 4-5 Glasses of Water per Day

You've heard for a very long time about drinking enough water—8 glasses per day or however much the prevailing wisdom is.

The truth is that there is no exact amount of water you're supposed to drink every day. If you're small and don't exercise much, then you need much less water. If you're big and extremely active, then you need a lot more.

This Big Win is not about how much water you drink, but rather when you drink it.

Drink:

1. 1 glass of water when you first wake up.

2. 1 glass of water immediately before each meal.

3. 1 glass of water just before bed.

If you eat 3 meals a day, that will be 5 glasses of water. If you skip a meal, it will be 4 glasses.

In an ideal world, you'd also drink water at other times (with and between meals), but not for this Big Win. The reason to drink water at these times is because it spaces out your water intake, helps remind you to drink more through the day, and also because drinking water in the morning and before meals helps to control how much you eat.

Above all else, drinking these glasses of water will often help you start to feel and think better and will improve your mood and outlook. Although that doesn't directly translate to weight loss, it often reduces the amount of food you eat because you get less stressed and less bored.

If you can create this habit in your life, it will help you achieve the Fundamental Principles of (a) automatically controlling hunger, (b) staying hydrated, (c) balancing your hormones, and (d) improving your mindset.

Summary

<u>4-5 Glasses of Water per Day</u>: This is a very easy Big Win, and as you'll see in the Quick-Start Guide, it's one of the ones I suggest starting with. It doesn't sound like it will make a huge difference for your weight loss, but over time, it can add up to a lot. Drink 1 glass of water upon waking, 1 glass before each meal, and 1 glass before bed.

Big Win #3: 35+ Grams of Protein for Breakfast

Remember that 3 of the Fundamental Principles are (a) automatically controlling hunger, (b) optimizing your hormones, and (c) improving your mindset. This Big Win covers all 3.

How to do it: Eat at least 35 grams of protein every morning for breakfast.

In other words, no matter what else you eat or don't eat, your breakfast must include at least 35 grams of protein. Here are some examples of what 35 grams of protein might mean:

- 5 ounces of lean beef or chicken;
- 6-7 eggs;
- 1-2 scoops of protein powder.

For example, you can have an omelet with some chicken and spinach in it or a green smoothie with protein powder.

The science behind this particular Big Win is impressive. Several studies have found that eating this much protein in the morning can dramatically reduce the amount of food that you eat overall during the day, can stabilize your blood sugar, and can reduce hunger and snacking.

The best part about this Big Win is that it's a habit you build first thing in the morning, and then you don't need to think about it for the rest of the day. At first, this will seem like a lot of protein, but after you get into the habit, it's incredibly easy to do.

Plus, you will likely stop eating as many carbs for breakfast just because you're eating so much protein. And eating fewer carbs in the morning will also give you more energy, help control your hunger, and make you feel better all day.

Summary

<u>35+ Grams of Protein for Breakfast</u>: Don't underestimate how powerful this one change can be. Make sure to eat 35 or more grams of protein every morning, and you'll feel fuller, happier, and more energetic all day long.

Slightly Less Pressing Food Concerns

As I mentioned at the beginning of this book, I haven't included anything that I don't believe is absolutely necessary. Still, there are quite a few moving parts.

When you work on the food that you're putting into your body, your first concern should be the 3 Big Wins. Those Big Wins will help you feel much better, and they'll make everything else you do easier.

Plus, I've seen many people make just 1 or 2 of those changes and start losing a lot of weight.

So if you're not doing those 3 Big Wins **consistently**, that's where you want to start. If you are already making those changes consistently, then here are a few Small Wins that might help you break through plateaus and lose more weight.

Small Win: No "Healthy" Versions of Junk Food

Even though this isn't a Big Win, I can't stress the importance of this Small Win enough.

When Louise and I first started eating Paleo, we tried to recreate everything from bread to cupcakes to cookies. As an occasional treat, that's not necessarily bad for your health.

But it's bad for your weight loss. One of the biggest problems with modern food is what's called "hyper-palatability." What that means is that if you combine a certain amount of sugar, fat, and salt into a single food, the human body becomes addicted to it. No matter if you're full, you can't stop eating.

Some people have more trouble with hyper-palatable foods than other people, but if you're overweight, then it's likely you fall into the camp that has more trouble. What I call "Healthy" Versions of Junk Foods are any food that would normally be processed junk food, but that you can now make with "healthy" ingredients (like almond flour, for instance). When you make these types of foods, you're almost always recreating a hyper-palatable food—you just happen to be using slightly less toxic ingredients to make it.

These foods will cause you to overeat, and besides, they almost always have some sort of "healthy" processed sugar in them, so they violate Big Win #1.

Small Win: Food Sensitivities

Food sensitivities are one way in which you might be very different from the person sitting next to you. However, most people don't understand food sensitivities very well.

The most surprising thing about food sensitivities is that they come and go. If you exercise very hard, you might have more food sensitivities for an hour or 2 after that, because your body is in a more stressed state. And if you start healing your gut, then many of your old sensitivities will usually go away.

Food sensitivities are a Small Win because if you eliminate the most common inflammatory foods, then you also get rid of much of the inflammation in your body. Other food sensitivities can obviously make a difference, but to a smaller degree, especially for weight loss.

If you know that you have a sensitivity to a food, then it obviously makes sense to avoid it. Don't throw fuel on the fire by continuing to eat a food that makes you feel bad.

However, I am not a fan of testing for sensitivities in a lab. Those tests can show you big allergies, but they're ridiculously inaccurate.

What I suggest instead is this . . .

If you *THINK* that you are sensitive to a food, then eliminate it for 30-60 days (during a Dash). Then try eating it again. If you're very sensitive to that food, you'll notice a difference.

It might surprise you, but I sometimes eat white rice now. Surely that's not very nutritious, right?

It's true—white rice isn't particularly nutritious. But I eliminated all grains from my life for nearly 6 years. And after reintroducing rice on various occasions, I've been able to tell exactly how my body reacts.

As it turns out, white rice doesn't seem to cause me any problems at all. However, you'll almost never see me eat anything with wheat in it. I'm not allergic or even highly sensitive, but I definitely don't feel as good after eating wheat.

> **Note About Food Sensitivities**: For any food that you think *MIGHT* be an issue for you, commit to eliminating it for at least 30 days. Then have it again and see how you feel. You might even need to repeat the experiment 2 or 3 times, but eventually, you'll have a very clear idea of how different foods are affecting your body. Obviously, for any major food sensitivities that you already know about, you should avoid that food.

Small Win: Eat More Veggies

There are many ideas that mainstream media has gotten wrong over the years. Eating vegetables is not one of them.

The reason that this is a Small Win is really because it's hard for most people. If you're not already eating a lot of vegetables, then starting to do so often means a lot of changes. It means more cooking, new recipes, and even learning to like new foods.

You can do all of that over time. I never ate any vegetables as a kid, and now they're most of what I eat. But it took me 10-15 years of changing my diet to get to this point.

Vegetables are not only nutritious, they're vital for the health of your gut (Fundamental Principle #3). You can get fiber and resistant starch from other places, but vegetables are one of the best sources you can find.

As a general rule, I encourage you to make every meal you eat mostly vegetables (1/2-2/3). It's just a guideline, and it doesn't matter if some meals are more and some are less, but it will greatly improve your digestion, your gut health, and your ability to lose weight.

Personally, I like starting every morning with a green smoothie that is loaded with spinach, kale, or another green, leafy vegetable. It's quick, it's easy, and it's automated, so I never have to think about what I'm going to eat.

Small Win: Eat Enough Food

On a real-food diet, one of the biggest mistakes I see people make is that they frequently eat too little. This often happens because they remove a bunch of junk foods from their diet and then don't add back in enough real foods.

If you're eating too little, it causes 2 big problems:

(a) It's not sustainable. You can't keep eating 1,200 calories for the rest of your life. You probably can't even keep it up for a week. So what you're doing is programming in failure. Your diet is designed to fail at some point—you just don't know when.

(b) The other big problem is that it's stressful on your body. When you're eating significantly fewer calories than your body needs, your body goes into panic mode, thinking that there just isn't enough food around. This causes mild inflammation in your body, but more importantly, it tells your body to hang on to all the fat that it can, because that fat is going to help you survive a famine. Unfortunately, that's not the result you're looking for.

There are no hard and fast rules for how much to eat, and I generally suggest not counting calories. If you're eating all the right foods, then your body will know. If you do want to measure it though, then most women fall somewhere between 1,600-1,900 calories, and most men fall somewhere between 2,000-2,400 calories. Obviously, if you're very active, you'll need a lot more.

Remember, we're not trying to voluntarily limit that amount of food or calories you eat—your body should take care of that on its own. But you do need to make sure that you're getting enough at each meal.

Small Win: Stop Snacking

All of the Big Wins in this chapter will help a lot with snacking. Drinking enough water, eating protein for breakfast, and removing inflammatory foods will help you feel less hungry throughout the day.

Also, if you're eating enough at every meal, you really shouldn't need to snack.

However, snacking is usually more of a psychological issue than a hunger issue. When we feel bored or upset, snacking is usually the first thing that comes to mind.

The problem is that snacking decreases your "metabolic flexibility." Metabolic flexibility is a fancy way of saying that your body should be able to burn both carbs and fat for energy. For an hour or so after you eat, your body has a lot of carbs floating around in your blood, and your body should be able to turn those into energy. After that (until you eat again), your body should be able to use the fat stored in your body for energy.

However, many of us aren't able to convert fat into energy as well as we should be. And when that's the case, you get hungrier and less energetic between meals, which means that you burn less fat, you eat more food, and you use less energy.

Snacking is not necessarily the cause of poor metabolic flexibility, but it makes it much harder to get over it. When you're eating all the time, your body never has a chance to learn to burn fat between meals (because you've got carbs from your snacks). One way to get around this is to avoid snacking as much as possible.

One of the best ways to do this is to find a different activity like walking or reading to do instead of snacking. This way, you're actively replacing the habit instead of just trying to avoid it.

Small Win: Eat Only Meat, Seafood, and Veggies

My friend Chris Kelly is very fond of telling people who want to lose weight to just eat meat and veggies.

And I sympathize with him, because this is how I often eat. Many of my meals are a plate of sautéed vegetables with a little bit of meat.

However, it's hard to do at first, and I've only gotten to this point after many years of refining my diet. I actually LIKE eating mostly meat/

seafood and veggies now, but that wasn't the case until the past couple of years.

If you've got everything else in order, it usually helps to get rid of all grains, legumes (beans), and even all tubers (potatoes), and fruits, as well as all seed oils, which are highly inflammatory.

Non-gluten grains, legumes, tubers, and fruits aren't terrible for you, but they're generally lower in vitamins and minerals, and if you have any existing gut issues, then some of these foods can exacerbate those issues and cause more inflammation. Seed oils ARE terrible for you, but I include them here because it's better to focus first on processed sugar, gluten, alcohol, and dairy.

The biggest benefits of eating only meat, seafood, and veggies are that you'll get lots of vitamins and minerals, you'll almost never eat too much, and you'll usually always get enough veggies.

Small Win: Eat the Same Foods Every Day

One of the best ways to automate your health and avoid slipping up or cheating is to eat the same foods every day. Eat the same meal for breakfast from one day to the next, the same meal for lunch, and the same meal for dinner.

The point is not to never diverge. Eating a different meal is fine. But having the routine in place makes your life and weight loss so much easier.

However, 99% of people hate this suggestion. It sounds boring.

But, if you interview the 100 healthiest people you know—especially the ones who used to be out of shape and have now stayed fit for a long time—you will find that the great majority of them eat the same foods over and over again.

Until a hundred years or so ago, humans ALWAYS ate the same foods over and over again. I understand that you might not want to do it, but the question is how much do you want to lose weight?

Eating the same food over and over again means, for instance, that you're never tempted to eat an unhealthy breakfast, that you don't have to use willpower to decide what to eat, and that you've got one less thing to worry about.

Personally, I drink a green smoothie (greens powder, coconut milk, protein powder, fiber supplement) 99% of the time for breakfast. You don't necessarily need to drink this smoothie, but choose something and stick with it.

Small Win: Cook in Bulk

If you have a job with long hours, this is especially important.

The best way to do this is to take a couple hours every Sunday to cook and plan. That way, you'll have food ready when you come home every weekday, and you won't need to worry about getting takeout or delivery (which are almost never good choices).

The times I used to cheat the most were when I was tired and had worked a long day. I had no willpower left over to make a good decision. But once Louise and I started planning ahead and actually having plenty of leftovers around, that changed completely.

Not as Important Considerations

There are a few issues you might be wondering about regarding food. These are popular topics, but I haven't really touched on them . . .

1. **Organic.** I'm not going to say much about organic foods here, except that organic versus non-organic doesn't matter much for weight loss. I'm not contending that organic is or isn't good, but you can't switch from non-organic to organic cookies and expect to lose weight.

2. **GMOs.** Genetically Modified Foods are no different than Organics, in that they make almost no difference for weight loss. Regardless of your view on the health or harm of GMOs, it's not something you need to worry about for weight loss.

3. **Grass-Fed or Wild-Caught.** Grass-fed beef and wild-caught seafood have become very popular over the past few years, and it's very likely that they're both healthier than the alternatives. However, the difference is relatively small, and for weight loss, the difference is almost zero. Not something you need to worry about for weight loss.

4. **Calories and Quantity.** In Chapter 3, I talked about calories. In the simplest terms, calories matter, but they're not all that matters. Eating 2,000 calories of cake is not the same as eating 2,000 calories of broccoli and chicken.

Even though calories matter, I generally don't encourage you to count calories. It can be occasionally useful to do for 3-5 days, just to get an idea of how much you're eating, but it's not a long-term strategy for weight loss.

In general, there are 2 possibilities:

1. **You're Really Good at Controlling How Much You Eat.** If this is the case, then great. You don't need to worry about how much to eat, because you already control it well. You don't overeat or snack too much. And if you're overweight, then you know that overeating isn't the issue.

2. **You're Really Bad at Controlling How Much You Eat.** If this is the case, then you're not going to get better. You're human, and you're not built to count calories. I've done it, and counting calories works, but it's miserable and you can't do it for a long time.

What I'm saying is that you could keep trying to count calories or control portion size, but I've seen almost nobody make it work long-term for weight loss. So while it matters in theory, it rarely works in practice.

Chapter 7

EXERCISE & MOVEMENT

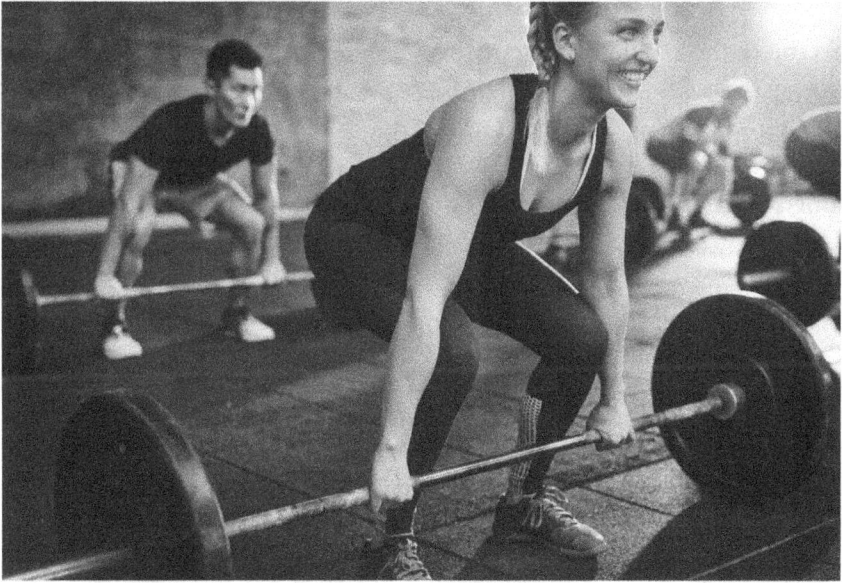

IN 2010, MIMI and Alex were busy planning their wedding.

At that time, Alex was working at a bank, and while he was home one evening, he overheard Mimi talking to her sister about the hair extensions Mimi had just bought for the wedding. Mimi was quite upset and felt like she had wasted a lot of money because the hair extensions were very low quality and didn't work the way she wanted.

Because of that experience, Alex and Mimi decided to create better hair extensions and start selling them themselves, all of which was fairly easy to set up. The problem was that Alex and Mimi had no way to market or advertise their product at that time.

What they decided to do was create a YouTube channel with tips on hair styling and other hair topics. So starting in 2010, they started posting one video per week to their channel.

At first, their videos honestly weren't very good. The lighting was average, the scripts weren't amazing, and although the videos definitely offered value to viewers, there was nothing spectacular about the videos.

But Mimi and Alex kept at it. They kept recording and releasing a video EVERY SINGLE WEEK, and they never stopped. As of 2015, they have over 270 million views and over 2.3 million subscribers. And their business is doing exceptionally well.

I don't know if you're interested in starting a business or becoming a YouTube star, but even if not, there's something we can all learn here. And it's something you probably already know but need to be reminded of.

It's the small and consistent steps that make all the difference. The little things (and the basics) add up over time.

If Mimi and Alex had stopped recording and posting videos, their business would never have been where it is now. And they didn't see many results in the first year or so. It was only after they'd been consistent at posting videos for over a year that they started to see a big payoff.

If that's the case for business, it's even more true for weight loss and for health. You don't need to be perfect in order to lose a lot of weight. You just need to be consistent with the Big Wins.

And two of those Big Wins are related to exercise.

In this chapter, I'll show you exactly why you don't need to do any sort of crazy exercises and why you don't need to work out for 3 hours a day. Those approaches don't work in the long run.

Here are the 2 Exercise Big Wins that absolutely do work for weight loss . . .

Big Win #1: Walk 10,000+ Steps per Day

Of all the things your body was meant to do (other than eating, sleeping, and having sex), walking is near the top of the list.

Like any animal with legs, your body is designed to walk. Walking is a low-impact activity, so you typically don't experience many injuries. Walking is necessary to get you from place to place. And walking has surprisingly powerful health and psychological benefits.

Unfortunately, for the past 100 years or so, we've become an increasingly sedentary culture. You probably sit down most of the day to work, to eat, or for many other reasons. We often sit down to watch TV or play games. And we even sit in our cars when we move from place to place.

The harms of sitting all day cannot be understated. We develop back problems. We get less circulation to various parts of our body, including our brains, which leads to mood swings. And sitting is highly correlated with all sorts of diseases from colon cancer to heart disease.

But perhaps most importantly for you, **the more you sit, the less likely you are to lose weight**. You burn fewer calories, your metabolism slows down, and various processes in your body just don't work as well. Plus, because motion creates emotion, you'll be less happy when you're moving around less, and that makes it much harder to take care of yourself like you need to.

The solution, then, is to walk more. But how much?

There is no magic answer. Generally, for weight loss, you should walk and move around *as much as you can.*

However, I know that "as much as you can" is vague, and you need a goal. From my experience—both personally and with people I've helped lose weight—**10,000 steps per day is the minimum you should aim for.**

10,000 steps per day is entirely doable for almost anybody. It might seem like a lot at first, particularly if you're very out of shape and not used to it. And if you need a week or two to work up to 10,000, then definitely take the time.

But in the end, when you start a Dash for this Big Win, aim for 10,000 steps per day.

I also understand that it's hard when you have a job, but you need to find a way. Take walks in the morning, at lunch, and in the evening. Get up and walk around the office every 45 minutes, if you can.

The absolute best solution if you're lucky enough to have a job that allows it is to create a walking desk. It's fairly easy and cheap—I created my first walking desk by putting some boxes on top of a table and then buying a $200 treadmill that would fit underneath the table.

Again, I'm not saying that incorporating a lot of walking into your day is easy for everybody. But it's necessary.

For measurement, you can either estimate your steps or else buy a device (like a FitBit) to track. Here are some estimates for how many steps you might be walking:

Walking Slowly: 75 steps/minute

Walking Moderately: 110 steps/minute

Walking Very Fast: 150 steps/minute

So it's likely that 10,000 steps will take you somewhere around 1.5-2 hours of walking.

Summary

10,000+ Steps per Day: Walk as much as possible, but aim for at least 10,000 steps per day during your Dash. Within just a few days, you will likely notice a range of benefits, including having more energy, a better attitude, and—of course—weight loss.

Big Win #2: Resistance Training 2 Days per Week

Even though you're interested in losing weight (particularly fat), you also need to think hard about preserving and/or building muscle and bone.

Muscle and bone are incredibly important for losing weight and keeping it off.

For instance, sometimes, you're going to eat more food than you burn. It's just going to happen.

In those situations, you want your body to use that food to build and repair bone and muscle tissue. The alternative is that your body will simply store that extra food as fat. However, your body won't use food for muscle and bone unless you give it a good reason.

As a plus, having more muscle will help you feel better and also to lose more fat.

Also, if you lose 20 pounds, you want most of that weight to be fat. You don't want to lose muscle and bone at the same time. Again, though, your body will lose muscle and bone unless you give it a reason not to.

And perhaps most importantly, having enough muscle is strongly linked to how healthy you are and how long you live. The science and research on this are very strong, and it's something discussed in more detail in Chapter 4.

What you'll need to do is to exercise in a way that shows your body that you need more muscle. That means doing things that are very hard for your muscles.

You don't need to do this type of exercise very often (2-3 times per week), and each workout should be pretty short (20-45 minutes). In fact, if you lift too often or spend too long doing it, you're not going to get all the benefits.

For this Big Win, you need to do **Some Sort of Hard Resistance Training 2 Days per Week.**

Here's a more detailed description:

- The exercise needs to be "hard" for you. This varies a lot from one person to another. The most important thing is that it needs to *feel* very hard for your muscles.

- This is not endurance exercise or cardio. It could include lifting weights, using machines that simulate weight-lifting, or doing bodyweight exercises like push-ups, squats, and lunges.

- Be safe, but push yourself. You need to give your body a reason to keep your muscle and bone. The only reason it will do that is if your body feels like you need the muscle and bone for hard physical activity.

If you have access to a gym and someone to show you how to lift weights, then lifting weights is one of the best solutions. Here's what I would recommend:

Day 1: Back Squat (5 sets of 5 reps); Bench Press (5 sets of 5 reps)

Day 2: Deadlift (5 sets of 5 reps)

For each set, you'd use the same weight, and if you can do all 5 sets, then you raise the weight slightly next time.

If you don't know how to do these exercises, then I highly recommend finding someone to show you. *Safety is the absolute most important thing, and you should NEVER lift without close to perfect form.* It's not worth it.

If you're not comfortable or familiar with lifting weights, then machines or bodyweight exercises will also work. By "machine," I mean machines in the gym that mimic lifting weights, not elliptical machines, stationary bikes, or treadmills. "Bodyweight" means exercises like squats, push-ups, and lunges.

The point is to work your muscles in a way that's difficult.

By the way, these types of exercise are extra-important if you're a little bit older. As you get older, it's easier to lose muscle and therefore more important to give your body a reason to keep it.

Again, this is Big Win #2 because lifting weight can really help ensure that the weight you lose is fat and not muscle or bone.

One final note . . . Don't worry that you're suddenly going to get big and bulky—I've never seen that happen by accident. It's a common fear, but the reverse almost always happens—doing resistance training makes you look and feel leaner rather than bulkier.

Summary

Resistance Training 2 Days per Week: For this Big Win, do some sort of hard resistance training at least 2 days a week. This could be lifting weights, using machines, or doing bodyweight exercises. The point is to push your muscles hard enough so that you don't lose but hopefully build bone and muscle.

Small Win: Sprinting

Apart from walking and resistance, the last great type of exercise your body needs is doing something very intense—something that will leave you breathing hard and tired from just a short workout.

I call this type of workout "sprinting," because the most popular form is to sprint (i.e., run really fast). However, it could be anything. You could run, swim, bike on a stationary bike, row if you have a rowing machine, do jumping jacks, or anything else, so long as 20-40 seconds of the activity is as much as you can do.

Here are general requirements for "sprinting":

1. Just one time per week.

2. 4-6 "sprints" on that one day.

3. Each "sprint" should be 20-40 seconds. You should not *be able* to do any more than that. After 20-40 seconds, you should be breathing really hard.

4. Between each "sprint," rest 1-2 minutes to catch your breath.

Here's the big caveat to all this. If you haven't done this sort of exercise in a long time, then **please be careful**. It's easy to injure yourself if you're not used to it, so take it slowly at first. And if you have some sort of illness or condition that might make it dangerous, obviously consult your doctor or healthcare professional first.

Resistance training and "sprinting" might not be fun or comfortable for you. But I wouldn't have included even this Small Win if it weren't beneficial.

Remember, though, that the Big Wins—like walking—are always more important. Don't try to do too much. Focus on 1-2 Big Wins per Dash, and you'll find that over time, you start to develop a lot of great habits and lose weight by accident.

Often, if you've got everything else in place, then lifting weights or sprinting can make a big difference. So please don't let a little bit of initial discomfort keep you from working these things into your life.

Small Win: Schedule Walks and Workouts with Friends

Whatever walking and/or resistance training you do, put it in your calendar/schedule with friends or family.

That way, you don't decide each day whether you're going to exercise or walk. It just happens at a particular time.

You might decide to skip an appointment one day. That's definitely a possibility.

However, if you keep doing it most of the time at that time, and if you schedule with another person, then eventually it will become habitual, and you won't even think about it anymore, much like you probably don't think at all about your drive to work.

Not as Important

Cardio

I need to say a word about cardio.

If you love running, elliptical machines, swimming long distance, or anything else that is typically considered "cardio," then that's fine.

But be absolutely clear—that's not an activity that you *need* to do in order to lose weight. In fact, in many situations (if your body is inflamed or stressed in other ways), then cardio can make it harder to lose fat.

I'm not telling you not to do cardio if that's what you want to do. But you don't need to.

Chapter 8

SLEEP

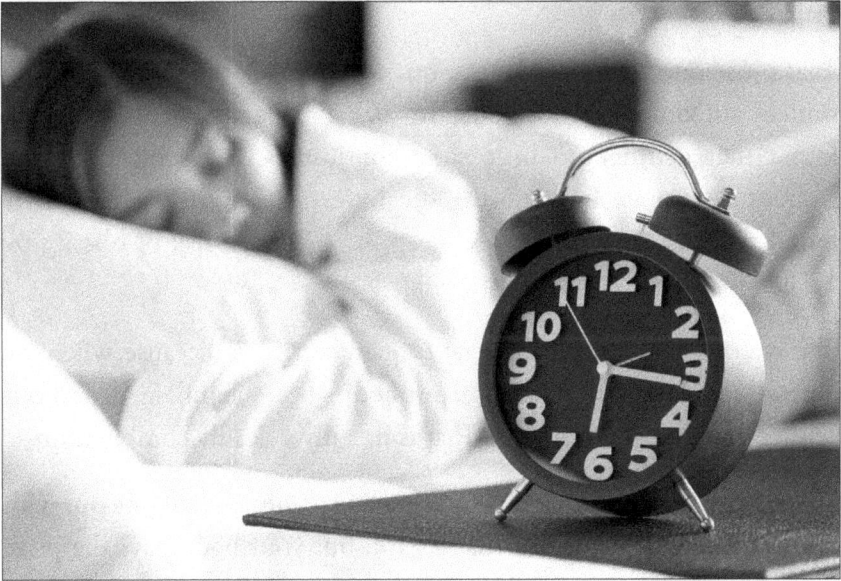

IN 2013, RESEARCHERS in Philadelphia, Pennsylvania gathered 225 people to run a sleep experiment. The experiment was only going to be a week, and the researchers were interested in seeing how sleeping more or less would affect weight gain.

197 of the participants were required to be in bed for only 4 hours for 5 nights during the week. The other 28 participants were allowed to be in bed for 10 hours every night during the week. And that's all that the researchers controlled. They didn't tell anybody what to eat, how much to exercise, or anything else.

After just one week, the 197 people who'd slept too little had gained an average of 2 pounds, while the people who slept enough had gained none.

Let that sink in for a moment. This is after just 5 nights of sleeping too little.

That's just one study, of course, but the number of studies showing similar outcomes is enormous. In 2011, researchers in New York found that getting too little sleep for just 2-3 days increased the amount people ate by almost 300 calories, and in 2015, researchers found that just 30 minutes less sleep increased the risk of obesity by 17%.

The reasons that sleep causes us to gain weight is because when we don't sleep enough, we eat more, our bodies become inflamed, and our cells become insulin resistant. That is literally a deadly combination.

We all love to stay up watching TV, playing games, or hanging out with friends. You're not alone in that regard, but your body pays the price in the end, and losing weight is almost impossible if you're consistently getting too little sleep.

Here is 1 Big Win and several Small Wins that will absolutely help you lose weight . . .

Big Win #1: 9 Consistent Hours in Bed in the Dark

The biggest win you can get with sleep is simply to consistently get enough of it. And there are so many obstacles to this . . .

- Work that needs to be done at night.

- Kids that don't sleep through the night.

- Not being able to go to sleep or stay asleep.

- Needing to check Facebook or watch another Netflix episode.

I'm joking a little, but I understand because I still struggle sometimes with consistently getting enough sleep. And no matter who I'm helping to lose weight, they rarely get enough sleep.

In fact, in one study, participants were put into a dark room for 14 hours per night. For the first 4 weeks, participants slept an average of *12 hours per night.* After the 4th week, they started sleeping an average of *8 hours per night.* That's how much sleep they needed to catch up on.

And you are likely no different. So getting 2-3 good nights of sleep is not going to be enough for you.

For this Big Win, you need to *consistently* be in bed in the dark for 9 hours per night.

There may be nights—especially at first, when you don't sleep for all or even most of that 9 hours. That's fine. The point is not only to get more sleep but also to develop a consistent routine.

If you start lying in bed for 9 hours in the dark every night, then your body will start to adjust, and you'll gradually start to sleep better and more. But it must be dark. You can't have the TV on or be working on the computer for part of this 9 hours. Otherwise, your brain won't adjust to the schedule, and you won't get the sleep your body needs to lose weight.

Many people ask me why 9 hours? The answer is that it's long enough to allow almost anybody to start catching up on sleep, and it's not so long that you'll feel like you can't do it. And everybody needs at least 8 hours of sleep per night.

No—you're not the one person on earth who only needs 5-6 hours of sleep. That might be what's normal for you, and you might be able to stay alive with that little sleep, but you're not at your best, and you won't be able to lose weight as easily.

Look, I've read tons of research on sleep, and I've talked to some of the smartest and most renowned sleep researchers in the world. It's true that how much sleep a person needs varies from one person to another, and it varies based on what you're doing during the day. (If you're incredibly active, you typically need more sleep.)

But sleep is integral for every human, and if you're not getting at least 7.5 hours per night, you are definitely sleep-deprived.

When you miss out on sleep, your body becomes inflamed, and the part of your brain that directs your self-control gets less glucose delivered to it. Being inflamed generally makes you hungrier and makes it harder to lose weight, and having less glucose delivered to the self-control portion of your brain means that you won't make good eating decisions.

And that's just the tip of the iceberg. You'll also quickly become insulin and leptin resistant, and you're much more likely to develop adrenal fatigue or start hosting pathogens in your gut (since your immune system won't be up to par).

I slept too little for the great majority of my life, and my body paid the price for it. When I got serious about losing weight, this made all the difference for me personally.

Summary

<u>9 Consistent Hours in the Bed in the Dark</u>: I've seen dozens of people be unable to lose weight AT ALL until they start getting enough sleep. Don't be one of them. For this Dash, set aside 9 hours per night to be in bed in the dark. Don't worry if you don't sleep the entire time—just create the routine.

Small Win: End the Party Early (Get to Bed Earlier)

I've always been a night owl, and my bedtime gets later and later if I let it. I like staying up late.

But that's one of the worst things you can do if you really want to lose weight, for 3 reasons:

1. You're occasionally (or frequently) going to need to get up early, so going to bed late just ensures that you'll get too little sleep on occasion.

2. If you don't keep a consistent bedtime, then your circadian rhythm (your internal clock) gets thrown off. When that happens, your body becomes more stressed, leading to extra inflammation and weight gain.

3. Finally, going to bed late is highly correlated with weight gain, obesity, and diabetes. In one study of over 1,600

people in Korea, the later you went to bed, the more likely you were to be overweight and diabetic.

So what does it mean to go to bed at a reasonable hour?

For the most part, it helps to be awake when the sun is up, which means that you'll want to get up around 6, 7, or 8 am, depending on the time of year and where you live in the world.

For that reason, you should usually be in bed by at least 10pm if not 9pm. I know that sounds incredibly early, especially if you still consider yourself to be young. However, it wasn't until I made this a priority in my life (only a few years ago) that I really stopped struggling with weight gain. And it's the same for many people I see succeed.

Small Win: Complete Darkness

In the Big Win for this chapter, I discussed darkness a bit. But if you want to see even better results, create a sleeping environment where you have zero artificial light. Even the smallest amount of light (from a streetlight, phone, or alarm clock) can actually cause you to lose sleep. And you won't usually realize it.

In addition, avoid artificial light for 2 hours before bed. For most people (including myself), this seems impossible, but it's not. Two hours before bed, commit to turning off all TVs, computers, phones, and fluorescent lights.

Ideally, you'd probably turn off ALL lights, but that's usually asking too much.

If you can't turn off all electronics at least an hour before bed, then the next-best option is to buy a pair of blue-blocking glasses (see here:

http://paleomagazine.com/amazon-blue-blocking-glasses), which are usually less than $10. These glasses will block out most of the blue light spectrum, which is the part that makes your brain think it's daytime. This will allow your brain to power down and get ready for sleep.

Not as Important

Sleeping enough and at the right times is critical. As with any chapter in this book, the Big Win is the most important piece.

However, in addition to the Big Win and the 2 Small Wins, here are a few other things to consider.

Note: You might have trouble sleeping well. Maybe you don't fall asleep well or you wake up often. I'm going to give you a couple tips to help with that, although these are not the only tips you might need. Sleep trouble can be caused by a variety of factors, some of which are entirely psychological, so it's impossible to give a complete list of solutions.

1. **Get Sunlight First Thing in the Morning**. Remember that you should ideally be getting up around the same time as the sun. As soon as you can, get out in the sun for at least 10 minutes. The sunlight on your eyes will wake your brain up and start to reset your circadian rhythm, which is vital to your sleep quality.

2. **Exercise, but Early in the Day**. Exercise is fantastic for improving your sleep quality, and I wrote a lot about exercise in the previous chapter. But whatever exercise you do, make sure it's earlier in the day. If you do it at night, it can easily disrupt your sleep quality.

3. **No Alcohol, Especially at Night**. Hopefully, you're already doing this. If you're not, then just know that alcohol is one of the things that disrupts sleep the most. It often helps you to fall asleep, but the sleep quality that you get is terrible. Ideally, you won't drink alcohol at all, but if you do, drink it earlier in the day. Nothing disrupts your sleep more than having alcohol in the evening.

Chapter 9

SUPPLEMENTATION

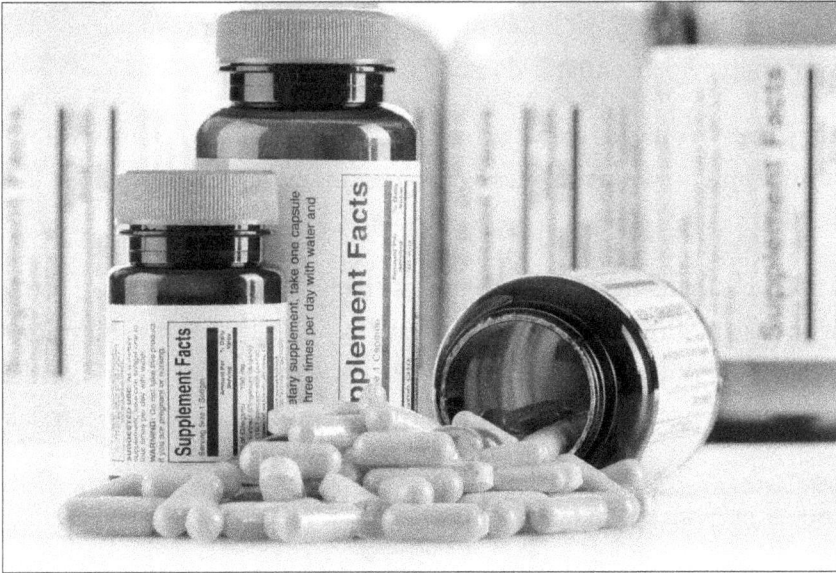

SOME ESTIMATES SAY that the supplement industry is worth $36 billion per year. Regardless of whether or not that number is correct, it's clear that the supplement industry is huge.

And it's no surprise. We all love the possibility of taking a few pills and having them change our lives and our bodies.

I have a 'supplement graveyard' at my house, where I've bought hundreds of supplements and never finished using them all. And I know I'm not the only one.

But with the rise of the internet, one thing is true. If any supplement were able to consistently cause weight loss, then you would hear about it EVERYWHERE. And that supplement alone would sell out overnight.

The fact that you don't know of any magical weight loss supplement is very good evidence that it doesn't exist.

In general, you can live an extremely healthy (and slim) life without any supplements at all. It's what humans have done for about 2.5 million years.

However, there are two supplements that can *potentially* help greatly with your health and weight loss. I say "potentially" because they don't make a big difference for every single person who takes them. For the majority of people, though, these supplements make weight loss much easier.

That's why there is only One Big Win for Supplements . . .

Big Win #1: 60 Days of Probiotics and Prebiotics

They say that the key to a man's heart is through his stomach. It's cheesy, but it's even truer that the key to anybody's health is through their stomach.

In particular, the microorganisms (bacteria, fungi, protozoa, etc.) that live in your gut have an enormous influence on your health. It's one of the 8 Fundamental Principles, and much of modern science is starting to show that this may actually be the biggest and most important principle.

In Chapter 11, I'm going to show you how to potentially get rid of any bad critters in your gut. But it's perhaps more important to actually support the healthy bacteria in your gut.

There are trillions of bacteria and other micro-organisms that live inside of you, and in some ways, they're actually more important for your health than your "human" cells. These bacteria help you digest food, they help fight off other infections, and they help your immune system to function properly.

STUDY: In some of the most impressive experiments ever, scientists have actually taken the gut bacteria from skinny mice and put that bacteria into fat mice. Within a week—without any other changes—the fat mice lost a bunch of weight. And this type of experiment has been repeated many times.

The moral of this story is that the bacteria in your gut is more important for your weight loss and health than you probably know. So what you need to do is make sure that you're (a) putting a lot of good bacteria into your body and (b) helping them to grow and thrive.

We don't know what a perfect gut would look like—or even if there is such a thing as a perfect gut. But we do know that it needs certain bacteria and other microorganisms, such as Bifidobacterium and Lactobacillus. You don't need to know or remember which bacteria are important for your gut. Just being aware is a good first step.

Eating a great (non-inflammatory) diet is the best and most necessary first step toward healing and improving your gut. So if you haven't implemented the Big Wins from Chapter 5, then you should definitely start there.

In addition, though, the following 2 supplements can give you another Big Win:

1. A Good Prebiotic Fiber.

2. A Good Probiotic.

Probiotics are the bacteria and other microorganisms that live in your gut and help your body to do all sorts of things, like breaking down food and fighting off illnesses. Prebiotics are the main food that probiotics eat (mostly in the form of fiber).

When you implement this Big Win in a Dash, I recommend that you do it for at least 60 days, first thing every morning. You can take both as capsules or along with a protein shake or smoothie.

It's an easy Big Win to implement, and your gut takes time to heal and change. 60 days is a good amount of time to do that.

For the prebiotic fiber, the easiest suggestion I can give is to use Prebio Plus: http://amzn.to/2baF2tZ. This prebiotic fiber is not perfect, but it's the best I've seen so far.

Although it's certainly possible to get enough resistant starch and fiber from foods, it's much easier to get them from these very inexpensive supplements. And why not? They're still derived from whole foods, and there are practically no side effects (other than a bit of bloating at first).

For the probiotic, my recommendation is Prescript-Assist (http://amzn. to/2bu785m). This is one of the few brands that both I and many other experts trust for both ourselves and everyone we recommend it to. In particular, it's got a great blend of "soil-based" bacteria, which are some of the most beneficial and most commonly missing bacteria from your gut.

One Final Note: If you're just starting to take probiotics and prebiotic, you might experience some initial discomfort, such as bloating and gas. This is natural to a degree, and most people get over it within the first week. However, if the symptoms persist, you might need to cut back on the prebiotic and work your way up more slowly.

Summary

60 Days of Probiotics and Prebiotics: Commit to 60 days of healing and optimizing your gut bacteria with one of the easiest Big Wins. Every morning, take a round of probiotics and prebiotics as soon as you wake up.

Additional Notes on Supplementation

In general, supplements get a bad rap. But there are also some good reasons that people think badly of supplements.

First of all, the supplement industry is more than a little bit shady. It's not well regulated, and many supplements are not high quality.

Perhaps more importantly, though, most people take supplements for very general reasons. Most people think a particular supplement will cure a particular ailment or will make them feel dramatically better. That's rarely the case.

With that in mind, there are a few things you should keep in mind with regard to supplements and weight loss:

1. **As of Today, "Weight-Loss" Supplements Do NOT Work.** There are no weight-loss supplements on the market that actually have any proven track record. So even if something seems to work for somebody, it's either an exception to the rule, or else it's a coincidence. Obviously, I believe that some supplements (like probiotics and probiotics) can help you lose weight. But that's not because they directly affect or cause weight loss. Rather, they have a big effect on your gut, which has big effects on the rest of your body.

2. **Supplementing for Known Deficiencies is Great.** If you have lab tests run that show a definite deficiency in a vitamin or mineral, then supplementing is usually the obvious course of action. For instance, if you're not getting enough Vitamin B12 for your brain to function properly, then by all means, supplement with B12. But guessing rarely works. Many people *think* they might be deficient in a vitamin or mineral, but they don't actually know. If that's the case, either get tested (see Chapter 11) or else let it go and don't supplement.

3. **Some Supplement Companies are Better than Others.** The list of bad supplement companies is too long to list. However, here is a very brief list of excellent supplement companies:

   - Klaire Labs

   - Thorne Research (perhaps the best overall)

- Designs for Health
- Douglas Labs
- Healthforce
- Life Extension

That's not a comprehensive list, but it's a good place to start. In particular, Thorne's standards are incredible, and I highly recommend them.

4. **Other Good Supplements**. Apart from prebiotics and probiotics, there aren't many supplements that everybody needs to take. However, a few that I often recommend are (i) a good greens powder—I like Amazing Grass, (ii) whey protein powder isolate—particularly for getting enough protein at breakfast, and (iii) magnesium—a mineral that almost everybody is deficient in.

5. **Elixa**. One supplement in particular—Elixa—deserves special mention. Elixa is a 6-day probiotic that is far stronger than anything else currently on the market. It also uses capsules that don't break down as easily, so the probiotics make it further into your gut. Combined, these 2 factors make Elixa a great option to use from time to time in order to repopulate your gut bacteria. You can order Elixa at http://www.elixa-probiotic.com.

6. **Eat More Fermented Foods**. This is not really a supplement, but it's strongly related to your gut health. Fermented foods include Kimchi, Sauerkraut, Kombucha, Natto, Kvass, and many others. Fermented foods are made when either yeast or bacteria turn the sugar in a food to alcohol. (Wine is also fermented, but I don't recommend it for these purposes.)

Fermented foods contain probiotics themselves, but they also contain "pre-biotics", which is what probiotics feed and live on. This means that the probiotics you eat in fermented foods are likely to live longer and actually make it into your gut.

Chapter 10

STRESS

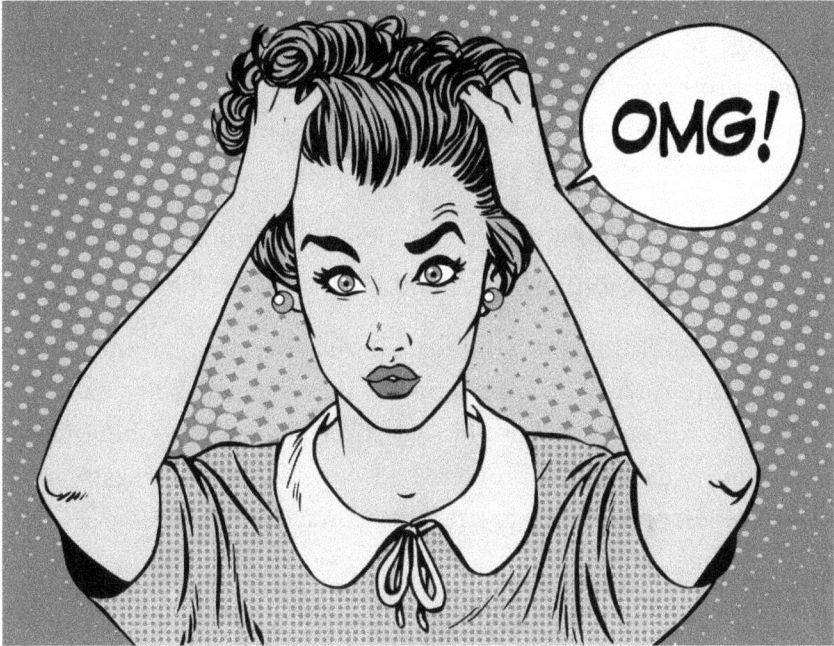

Aᴛ ᴛʜᴇ Wʀɪɢʜᴛ brothers built and flew their first plane in 1903, they had a bit of a honeymoon for the next 8 years.

They continued to work extremely hard, but everything started going very well for them. Their planes just got better and better, and everyone from the US government to French businessmen started to buy their airplanes. They were world-famous and generally enjoying it.

But by 1911, several things changed for the brothers. Most of their business was based in shows, where pilots would fly their planes faster, higher, and in death-defying stunts. And that put a great deal of pressure on Wilbur and Orville, partially because many of their pilots were dying during these shows.

In addition, several people around the world were trying to take advantage of their success by filing huge patent lawsuits against the Wright brothers. This meant that the brothers had to spend a lot of time in court and with lawyers, trying to hold on to the business they had created.

All in all, life was not nearly the joy-ride it had been. And in 1912, it took a more tragic turn when Wilbur contracted Typhoid and died.

Stress is an incredibly powerful force in our lives, and it's one that we often underestimate. It's quite possible that Wilbur's body was more susceptible to illness because he was stressed. But more importantly, even though the Wright brothers had done so many things right in their business and life, it was stress that unraveled everything.

Dr. Sapolsky, a professor at Stanford, has studied stress extensively, often in African baboons, who have very similar social structures and lives to humans. What he and other researchers have found is that stress is very highly linked to almost every chronic disease that you could name: heart disease, cancer, fatigue, depression, hypertension, digestive issues, and much more.

And perhaps most importantly, *psychological stress almost always leads to weight gain, usually around the belly*. Stress has a direct effect on our gut bacteria, it creates inflammation in our bodies, and it makes us fat.

Your Stress Level is Higher than You Think

Unless you're actively managing your stress, it's quite likely that you have a lot more stress in your life than you think you do.

If you feel like parts of your life are out of control. Or if you feel like you "must" do certain things in your life or every day. Or if you feel like some things in your life are getting worse.

Those are all feelings of stress, and in our modern world, these feelings are much more the norm than the exception. While so much of our lives is getting better and healthier, stress is one of the few areas of our lives that seems to be getting worse in many ways.

When I talk to people about their health, I can often get them to eat better, to exercise, to sleep more, and I can even convince them that they should do more lab testing. But I find that I have the hardest time getting people to deal with the stress in their lives.

Even if we acknowledge that we're stressed, we often accept it as the way things are or else we don't believe we can actually eliminate our stress. And I'll be the first to admit that I still struggle from time to time with stress.

But it can get much better, and if you want to lose weight, then you *need* to deal with some of the stress in your life.

There is no magic formula for dealing with stress, but there are a few things that I see help people time and again.

Big Win #1: Meditate for 10 Minutes per Day

Meditation is—for some reason—controversial. But I don't really understand why.

You don't need to believe in anything in particular or be religious at all to experience the benefits of meditation. More to the point, there are now thousands of studies showing the health benefits of meditation, and those benefits extend far beyond weight loss to other aspects of our lives.

Often, I hear from people that meditation just doesn't work for them, or that they can't get their mind to stop racing. But that's not the point—meditation is not a game where the goal is to quiet your mind. That often happens, but it's really just a side-effect.

The point of meditation is to become more aware of your thoughts, and that's it. You'll experience other benefits (reduced stress most of all), but the sole point is to gradually become more aware.

If you haven't meditated before and want an easy way to get started, then I recommend an App called "HeadSpace." You can find it on either the Apple App Store or on the Google Play App Store. It's free to use (for a while), and it's the easiest way I know of to jump into just 10 minutes of meditation per day.

Obviously, if you want to go more in depth, then there are many websites and even local meditation centers where you could learn more. However, I'm not encouraging that you become a monk and start meditating for hours per day. Just 10 minutes a day will do a world of good for your stress levels, and once you get your stress levels down, weight loss becomes amazingly easier.

Summary

<u>Meditate for 10 Minutes per Day</u>: Meditation is not *essential* for weight loss. Many people have lost weight without ever meditating. However, reducing your stress levels is absolutely necessary, and meditation is the best and easiest way to do that.

Small Win: Walking, Sun, & Nature

Our brains are wired from millions of years of evolution to react well to "nature," sun, and the outdoors. For patients in hospitals, several studies have found that even pictures of the outdoors help reduce stress and increase recovery rates.

You probably aren't in a hospital, and you might think that you don't like nature or the outdoors. That's fine, but you still need to get outside, because there are few things that will destress your body and mind more effectively.

Walking, in addition to being great for your body and hormones, is also excellent for reducing stress. So to the degree possible, whenever you incorporate walking into your day, try to walk outside—at least in the sun, but preferably in a non-urban setting.

When I used to work in Manhattan, New York, I would walk every day during lunch through Central Park. It wasn't wilderness, but then I don't really love the wilderness, and Central Park still gave me sun, trees, grass, and plenty of space to walk in.

In addition to walking, just getting outside to play, to garden, or to sit, are all great ways to help alleviate stress. And don't wait until you "feel" stressed. The point is to do these activities frequently and often, because we often have low levels of stress that we don't even acknowledge. If you work these activities into your daily life, then stress will start to disappear before you ever notice it.

I know that this might be one of the practices in this book that you find most disconnected from losing weight. After all, everything we've ever been told is that what we eat and how much we exercise are the cornerstones of weight loss. And to be sure, they're both very important, which is why I included chapters in the book dedicated to diet and exercise.

But stress is no less real. And it WILL prevent you from losing weight, even if you don't think you're stressed out.

Getting outside more often is the simplest and easiest way to start to relieve some of that stress, so please don't overlook this practice.

Also, find ways to play in the dirt again. Many of the most important bacteria we need as humans come from the soil. And that was easy when we all used to live on dirt, play in the dirt, dig for food in the dirt, and farm in the dirt. Now, however, many of us never come in contact with the soil.

Small Win: Random Stress Thoughts

In general, most of the stress in our lives comes from what I call Life Incongruence.

That's my fancy way of saying that certain parts of our lives often don't match up with the way that we feel they should be. We think our spouse isn't loving enough. We don't really like the city we live in. Or we hate going to our job every day.

In any of those situations, we feel a constant underlying stress because we have a desire for things to be different. Unfortunately, we often don't take any action to make things different because we either feel like things are out of our control or else we're too scared of making big changes.

Nobody in the world is immune to these sorts of problems. However, the happiest and healthiest people find ways to take action anyway. If you're not happy in your job, you need to find a way out or else figure out how to make it something you love. I know all the excuses— what else would I do, I have people to support, etc. But they're all just excuses.

Whenever we really want something in our lives, we're ALL capable of going out and getting it. There's going to be discomfort along the way, but if we commit ourselves, anything is possible.

The point is that you can't let these things fester for the rest of your life. Deep down, you know which parts of your life are not fulfilling for you. You may not know what the answer is, but you need to start taking some sort of action in those areas, even if it makes things worse at first.

Unlike most of this book, I can't offer you any advice on specifically what action to take, partially because I don't know your situation, but partially because it doesn't matter. Once you start changing things, you'll figure it out, even if you head the wrong direction to begin with.

Most of this chapter probably seems only distantly related to weight loss, but I encourage you to start believing that your health and weight loss are not disconnected from the rest of your life. Usually, if one area of our life is in disarray, then several other areas are as well.

Chapter 11

LAB TESTING AND PATHOGENS

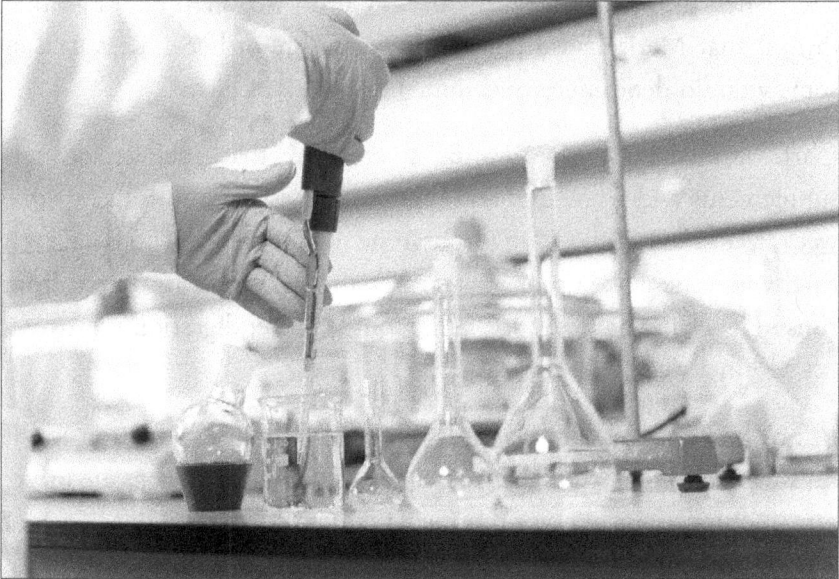

A LITTLE OVER A year ago, my friend Chris received a call from a woman named Maria. Chris helps people find and deal with the underlying causes of their health problems, from weight loss to fatigue to almost anything else.

Maria was 50 years old, worked with college athletes, and was very into sports. She loved running and being as active as possible. However, for quite a while, Maria had been feeling more and more exhausted and she needed longer to recover. She was eating well, exercising a lot, and believed that she was doing almost everything right.

She thought that maybe it was simply a sign of getting older, but when her hair started to fall out, she knew something was wrong.

Chris suggested that she run a few lab tests to help figure out what was going on in her body, and Maria immediately agreed. A few weeks later, when the test results came back, Chris discovered (among other things) that Maria had a parasite living inside of her gut, as well as some vitamin deficiencies and some hormonal problems.

Chris immediately gave Maria a protocol that included a few supplements and a few diet and lifestyle suggestions. Within just one week, Maria started sleeping through the night again, she no longer felt tired when she woke up or in the early afternoon, she recovered from runs quickly, her hair stopped falling out, and her digestion improved. All within a week.

I don't know if you can relate to Maria at all, but her situation is not unusual. You might think that parasites and other pathogens are pretty rare in our guts, or that you'd notice if you had a vitamin deficiency or a hormonal problem. But that couldn't be further from the truth. It's actually very common, and if you have any sort of health issues, then you more than likely have some sort of pathogen in your gut and some sort of deficiency.

Maria didn't actually need to lose any weight, but I've also seen many people heal the pathogens in their gut and start losing weight almost immediately. One police officer found after testing that he had a few pathogens and deficiencies. Within 60 days of being on a protocol to heal his gut (specific to his issues), he lost 26 pounds without eating less or exercising more (he was already eating a Paleo diet).

Your gut is the key to your overall health (as well as your weight loss). It's where your body is able to absorb every nutrient that you need, it's the part of your body that protects your bloodstream from bacteria and pathogens, and it's where most of your immune system is based.

It's also more than just parasites and pathogens. If you don't have the right balance of good bacteria in your gut, then you can't break down food properly, and you're much more likely to get sick.

In other words, if your gut is not working properly, then the rest of your body probably isn't either. But, for the most part, we don't take care of our guts like we should. In this chapter, I'll show you 1 Big Win you can take to figure out exactly what's going on in your body, address those specific problems, and also heal, rebuild, and optimize your gut.

The Big Win in this chapter often produces the biggest gains in weight loss in the shortest amount of time.

One Very Important Note

The tests I recommend below are not inexpensive and are not usually covered by insurance (especially in the US). I understand that these tests might be out of your budget.

Don't use this as an excuse not to implement the recommendations in the rest of this book. If you implement the rest of the Big Wins in this book (one or two-at-a-time through the Run then Rest System), you will almost certainly get great results.

In fact, in the Quick-Start Guide, I don't even include the testing because I know that many people can't afford it.

But I would also be remiss if I didn't alert you to the possibility and upside of this testing, because it really can change your body and life faster than almost anything else, depending on what sorts of underlying issue and pathologies you might have in your body.

Big Win #1: Get Tested

You might want to make just a few changes at home to your diet and lifestyle. It's easier, more comfortable, and frankly, less expensive.

But **I cannot emphasize enough how important it is to know exactly what's going on inside your body.**

Think about it. If you don't have enough CoQ-10, for instance, you're going to continually feel tired and sluggish. If you've got a C. Difficile infection, then you're going to be unable to lose weight and will get sick a lot more often. And if you are low on B12, your mood will almost never improve to where it should be.

These are all things that you could know very easily and fix within a few months, but only if you're willing to do the tests.

Below, I've listed 3 tests that I believe EVERYBODY should get. I personally try to get them once per year, but you should especially get them if you feel like you can't lose weight or you have some other health issue.

You can order these tests yourself at places like MyMedLab.com or LabTestsOnline.com, or you can have someone like my friend Chris Kelly (www.nourishbalancethrive.com) order and analyze the tests for you. He'll provide you with a personalized protocol and consultation once you get your results. You can also order them through many doctors and naturopaths, but you'll need to make sure they know how to interpret the results. If you prefer to work directly with someone, you can also reach out to me, and I will point you in the right direction.

And to be clear, I am NOT mentioning these tests in order to sell you anything. These tests are the only thing I recommend in this book that you buy (besides a very few probiotics and prebiotics). I'm recommending these tests because I've seen firsthand the difference they make for people, and it's incredible.

Many people can lose weight without these tests. But not everybody can, and more importantly, these tests can make it much faster and easier.

There are 3 tests, and you should get all 3, because they work together to tell you different things about your body. If you get just one, it might help, but you might not be addressing all of the underlying causes.

Test #1: DUTCH Hormone Test. (Order from Precision Analytical, Inc.—https://dutchtest.com/). The DUTCH Hormone Test will show you whether you're producing too little, just enough, or too much of certain hormones. Specifically, the test will show your levels of cortisol, DHEA (an anabolic hormone), estradiol and estriol (both of the estrogen family), testosterone, progesterone, and melatonin.

Hormones are the messengers of your body. Essentially, they tell every part of your body what to do and when. This test will allow you to support those hormones either through temporary supplementation or through temporary diet and lifestyle changes.

When it comes to weight loss, certain hormone problems are a huge issue. If you've got very low cortisol, for instance, losing weight is extremely difficult because it will affect both your thyroid and also your energy expenditure. Same if you have low DHEA, too little testosterone, or too much estrogen.

Test #2: Urine Organic Acids. (Order from Genova Labs). The Organic Acids Test is a comprehensive way to see whether or not certain processes in your body are working properly. Here's a list of just a few of the processes that an Organic Acids Test will tell you about:

- Fat burning
- Blood sugar stabilization
- Energy production
- DNA Methylation
- Toxins and detoxification
- Oxidative stress/antioxidants
- Neurotransmitter turnover
- Intestinal bacterial overgrowth

Apart from just the fat burning, you can see how important those processes are. For instance, if your energy production cycle isn't working properly, then you'll feel fatigued and you won't burn much energy. When each of these processes occurs (or doesn't occur properly), your body produces things called organic acids, and these organic acids can be measured in your urine.

Just imagine that you're driving on the freeway, and you notice that the check engine light is on. Do you automatically know what's wrong? Of course not. You need a mechanic to examine the car and plug in a computer to see what's going on.

Fatigue, foggy thinking, loss of libido, and even weight gain are the human version of the check engine light, and organic acids can reveal the causes. It's extremely rare (less than one in a hundred) to see results on this test without room for improvement, so it makes sense to do this test no matter what.

Test #3: Comprehensive Stool Analysis. (Order from Biohealth Labs). If you remember Maria from the beginning of this chapter, one of her biggest issues was that she had pathogens in her gut. The pathogens can take the form of bacteria, yeast, fungus, parasites, and other tiny critters. And when you have these pathogens, your body works overtime to get rid of them and can't focus on other things like weight loss.

In this test, various fancy techniques are used to identify bacteria and parasites that could be interfering with digestion, causing inflammation, and generally preventing you from getting better. Pathogenic organisms are one of the leading causes of fatigue and weight gain, but they almost always go unnoticed and untreated.

When you run this test, here's just a *short* list of what might come up:

- Cryptosporidium parvum
- Entamoeba histolytica
- Giardia lamblia
- Blastocystis hominis
- Endolimax nana
- Candida
- Helicobacter pylori
- Clostridium difficile

Truthfully, the microbiologist never knows what they're going to find. However, the upside is that once you do find something, it's fairly easy and quick to get rid of, meaning that your health will usually rapidly improve.

Summary

<u>Get Tested</u>: If you can afford it, get tested, and don't wait to do it. Other changes like diet and sleep will help, but if you have severe deficiencies or pathogens, then it's very hard for your body to fully recover.

Chapter 12

SECRET WEAPON FOR WEIGHT LOSS

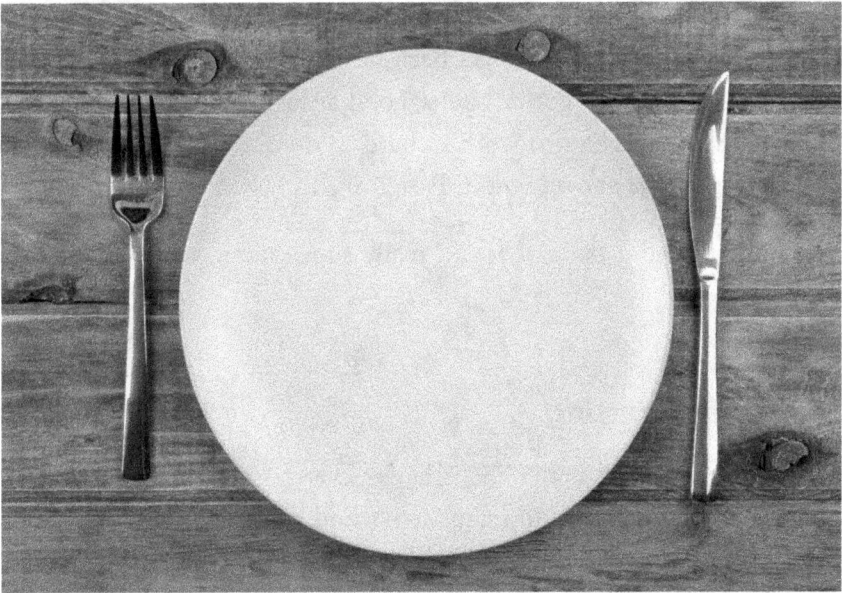

Throughout this book, I've shared other people's stories with you. I believe that stories are a great way to understand and relate to an idea.

For this secret weapon chapter, I want to share a bit more of my own story with you. You see, my story didn't really *end* a few years ago when I noticed that I was able to accidentally lose weight and keep it off.

Around May of 2015, I noticed that I'd let certain things slip. I was eating a little bit too much inflammatory food, I wasn't moving enough, and I was very stressed in general. As a result, I had regained some of the weight that I'd lost.

As you can imagine, I wasn't happy to admit all of this to myself. But I couldn't ignore the truth that my clothes weren't fitting as well as they used to.

So I made a commitment to get back in shape that summer. Over the course of my life, I've gotten pretty good at losing weight and getting in shape, since I've had to work so hard to do it. So I followed all the Big Wins that I've shown you in Part 2 of this book.

But I also added a piece that can really supercharge your weight loss results . . .

Intermittent Fasting

And my results were better than they've ever been. In 11 weeks (with one of those weeks off), I lost almost 5% bodyfat (around 16 pounds of fat). I measured using DEXA scans before and after the 11 weeks, and DEXA scans are the most accurate measurement you can get.

I'd done some intermittent fasting prior to that summer, but only occasionally. So I was very excited by my results.

However . . .

2 Warnings About this Secret Weapon

As much as I love intermittent fasting, I have 2 warnings about it.

1. Don't Start Here. If you're still eating a lot of inflammatory foods, not staying hydrated, or aren't sleeping enough, then intermittent fasting is NOT the place to start. You won't get the same results from fasting, and it might even be worse for your body.

Fasting is a potential source of stress on your body because your body thinks it's not getting enough food. Fasting is not a bad stress if your body isn't under a lot of other stress. But if you're not already applying the other Big Wins, then the potential stress of fasting could do more harm than good.

2. Easier than You Think. If you haven't fasted much in the past, then it sounds like a terrible and very painful idea. After all, you probably get hungry and angry after not eating for just a few hours. How will you feel if you go for 16 or 24 hours without food?

The answer is that it can be a bit tough at first, but it's never as tough as you think it's going to be. It's more about your mindset than anything else. You're used to eating all the time, and so it seems like it's going to be terribly uncomfortable.

If that sounds like what's going through your mind right now, then just relax. You don't have to try intermittent fasting if you don't want to. However, the vast majority of people who end up trying it also end up loving it.

The Benefits of Intermittent Fasting

The first benefit of intermittent fasting is obvious. You eat less, which means that weight loss is automatically easier. This doesn't need much explanation.

The bigger benefits, though, are that you (a) feel less hungry in general, (b) your attitude and mental clarity improve, and (c) fasting leads to "autophagy." This last effect is particularly important. Autophagy is the process by which the cells in your body recycle dead, diseased, or worn-out cells. (That's a simplistic description of a very complicated process.)

When you increase autophagy, a number of amazing things happen:

- Your average lifespan increases;
- Your risk of heart disease decreases;
- Your risk of cancer significantly decreases;
- Your body increases production of Growth Hormone, which allows you to build and maintain more muscle and bone;
- Your brain immediately starts functioning better, and your risk of neurological disorders decreases.

As you can see, intermittent fasting does a lot for your body other than just allowing you to eat less. And it's not surprising, since humans for almost 2.5 million years were forced to fast regularly, since they couldn't always find enough food.

However, these are all just the extra benefits. The biggest benefit for you is that weight loss is MUCH easier and more likely with intermittent fasting.

With that in mind, here are 2 different ways to use intermittent fasting as a secret weapon to dramatically increase your weight loss . . .

Big Win #1: Intermittent Fasting

Unlike all of the other Big Wins in this book, I'm going to show you 2 different options for this particular Big Win. Both options work very well, and it depends mostly on which you like best.

Option #1: Fast for 16-18 Hours Every Day.

This is the most popular way to do intermittent fasting. And honestly, it's not all that different from how you probably eat right now.

If you eat dinner at 8pm and eat breakfast at 7am the next morning, then you're already fasting for around 11 hours (assuming that you don't snack at night).

With this Big Win, all you would do is extend that time to 16-18 hours. In other words, if you eat dinner at 8pm, then you wouldn't eat again until 1 or 2pm the next day. Another way to think about it is to only eat during a 6-8 hour window each day. When you think about it this way, you would only eat between 1pm and 9pm, for instance.

This option still provides all the benefits of intermittent fasting, but it allows you to eat lunch and dinner just like normal.

Option #2: Fast for 36 Hours 1-2 Days per Week.

This option is less popular, but it's the option I prefer and that I see the best weight-loss results from. When I was losing weight in the summer of 2015, this was the way that I did it.

To do this, you simply choose 1 or 2 days a week that you want to fast. Then you don't eat at all that day. It turns out that you fast for around 36 hours, assuming that you eat around 8pm on the day before fasting and then around 8am on the day after fasting.

Start with 1 day per week and then move to 2 days per week once you get used to it.

Going 1 day without food sounds daunting, and it can be tough if you've got meetings or other activities that typically revolve around food. But if you can schedule fasting days when you don't have many social engagements, this can be incredibly effective.

No matter which option you choose, all there is to it is to simply not eat for either 16 or 36 hours. It's really that simple, and it's far easier and more effective than you might think.

Summary

Intermittent Fasting: Intermittent Fasting really is a secret weapon for weight loss and health. It's incredibly healthy and often kickstarts weight loss when you've hit a plateau and nothing else works. Choose either to fast for 16 hours every day or else for 36 hours 1-2 days per week, and go for it. But do this only once you've got most of the other Big Wins in place.

Chapter 13

SHORT LIST OF BIG WINS

IN CASE YOU need to reference them, here is the complete list of Big Wins for Weight Loss.

Remember, these are the actions that will help you most quickly and easily get all of the Fundamental Principles right in your life. But don't try to do them all at once—that will guarantee failure. In the next chapter, I'll explain the Run then Rest System in more detail, so that you can implement these Big Wins in a way that will last a lifetime and ensure that you're able to lose weight and keep it off.

1. Get Clear on Your Pain.

2. Hold Yourself Accountable.

3. Eliminate Inflammatory Foods (Gluten, Processed Sugar, Alcohol, & Dairy).

4. 4 Glasses of Water a Day (Upon Waking & Before Breakfast, Lunch, & Dinner).

5. 35+ Grams of Protein for Breakfast.

6. Walk 10,000+ Steps per Day

7. Resistance Training 2 Times per Week

8. 9 Hours in Bed in the Dark Every Day

9. Probiotics + Prebiotics

10. 10 Minutes of Meditation per Day

11. If You Can Afford It, Lab Testing as Outlined in Chapter 11.

12. Once You Have Everything in Place, Intermittent Fasting.

PART III

THE RUN THEN REST SYSTEM + QUICK-START GUIDE

Chapter 14

THE RUN THEN REST SYSTEM

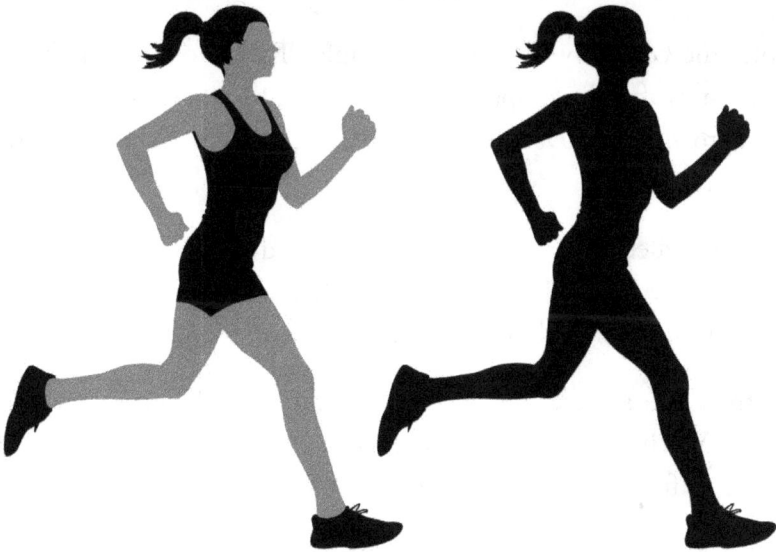

2,600 YEARS AGO, Aesop wrote a story that still captivates kids and adults everywhere.

In that story, a hare made fun of a tortoise for being slow, so the tortoise challenged the hare to a race. The hare raced ahead but then as a jest, decided to take a nap, thinking that he could catch up to the tortoise at any time.

However, the hare overslept and woke up only when the tortoise was about to cross the finish line.

The moral of this well-known fable is that "slow and steady wins the race." And it's widely accepted as wisdom for health, business, and many other areas of life.

However, the truth is that slow and steady **_usually doesn't_** win the race.

Apple (the company) is a good example. They're one of the biggest and most profitable companies in the world, but they didn't just chug along, growing by 10% every year. In fact, for much of the 1990s, they lost money.

But then, when they came out with the iPod and iTunes, everything changed very quickly for them. Sure, they had persistence and kept going, but it wasn't a slow and steady progress.

Health is the same. You don't treat a disease or injury slowly and steadily. You have surgery, you take aggressive drugs, or you make a big lifestyle shift.

And people who are successful at losing weight and keeping it off don't approach weight loss in a slow and steady manner. It's true in my own life and in the lives of _almost_ everybody I've coached or talked to about weight loss.

So if "slow and steady" isn't the way to lose weight, then what is?

The Run Then Rest System

In Part 2, I showed you the Big Wins that will help you start losing weight by accident. If this were a normal diet book, I'd give you a sample meal plan and tell you to go for it.

But you and I both know that doesn't work for most people, and it probably won't work for you.

Instead, you are going to use the Run then Rest approach. This is a tool that will allow you to get **quick and impressive results**. It will also allow you to **keep the weight off without dieting 100% of the time**.

Here's why it works . . .

Sticking to a Diet is the Hardest Part

Diets work. Cutting calories works. Exercise works.

If you could keep doing it.

Luckily, you are not forced to do anything. You can eat what you want, exercise if you want, and do whatever you like.

It's a blessing, but for weight loss, it's also a curse. To lose weight, you need to *voluntarily* force yourself to be healthy. And that's harder than ever with so many temptations readily available like addictive junk foods and Netflix to keep you from going to sleep or to the gym.

And because it's so hard, most people continually fail at dieting and exercise, even if they know what they should be doing.

Most importantly, your body and mind are not evolved to diet or exercise continuously for long periods of time.

The Basics of the Run then Rest Approach

Luckily, there's an alternative, and it's what I call the *Run then Rest System*. Here's how it works:

1. For a set amount of time (1-2 months), you do a "**Dash.**" During this Dash, you make 1-3 changes that will result in "Big Wins." I showed you all of these Big Wins in Part 2— these are the changes that are designed to be the domino that causes many other pieces to automatically fall into place.

2. Then, after the Dash, you take 1-2 months and take a "**Rest.**" You relax, but you automatically keep at least some of the good habits you built during the Dash.

3. And then you start the process again with a new Dash.

It's a simple process, but it works. It works because the human brain is capable of focusing and making a few changes at a time.

And in the next chapter, I'll outline the exact Dashes that I recommend to maximize your weight loss.

However, that doesn't mean that you couldn't design your own Dashes. Especially once you get in great shape, you might need to be more nuanced and advanced in the changes you make.

Here are the reasons why the Run then Rest System works, and also some traps to avoid falling into:

1. <u>Focus</u>: During a Dash, you make no more than 1-3 changes at a time. And you focus on those changes for 1-2 months. If you try to make more changes during that time, you'll fail. It's true for me and for everyone I've seen try it. You

can lose a lot of weight and make a lot of progress in 1-2 months, but only if you do less, rather than more.

2. <u>Big Wins</u>: The changes that I will give you to make are ones that make the biggest difference for your weight loss. These are the changes that will allow you to capture the 8 Fundamentals of weight loss (all of which I discussed in Chapter 4). If you make less important changes, then you might see some improvement, but likely not nearly as much.

3. <u>Rest</u>. This is huge. When you get motivated or inspired, you temporarily believe that you can do anything. But particularly with diet and weight loss, it's just not the case. Losing weight is actually stressful on your body, so your body needs time to adjust and recuperate. If you don't take the time off between Dashes, then you'll eventually fall off the wagon completely.

If it seems simple, that's because it is. Weight loss can be incredibly simple, and even accidental, if you do just a few things right. But you've got to do the right things, and you need to do them in a sustainable way.

The Run then Rest System is the most effective and sustainable approach you can take. But you've got to do the right things during a Dash, and the right things are the Big Wins I showed you in Part 2.

So What Do You Do During a Dash??

You **focus**. And that means 2 things:

1. **1-3 Changes**. You make between 1 and 3 changes to some area of your life. And the changes that you make should be

Big Wins (Chapter 13 has a full list of Big Wins). You don't try to do more than this . . . just 1-3.

2. **Strict**. During the Dash, you are very strict about those 1-3 changes. It's your entire focus, and nothing else should get in the way. Life happens, and you're not perfect, but you should try as hard as possible to be perfect about those changes.

3. **Track**. Every single day, you MUST track whether you made the changes you were supposed to. And you can't just do this in your head. You need to print out a calendar with the changes listed for each day (you can download a complete calendar based on the Chapter 15 Quick-Start Guide from http://jeremyhendon.com/accidental-weight-loss-calendar), and you need to hang it somewhere so you'll see it every day. Then you need to cross off each day when you successfully make those changes.

Other than that, you don't worry about anything else during the Dash. One Dash likely isn't going to be all you need. That's the whole point. By doing these Dashes, you're building up your health so that weight loss happens automatically and also stays off automatically.

And What Do You Do During a Rest??

This is an important question. One of the problems with most diets is that after you fall off the wagon, you go back to your old way of eating/living. And when you do that, you get your old body back (along with all the weight you might have lost).

That doesn't need to happen.

A lot of the reason people fall of the wagon completely is because they never gave themselves any room to breathe. The Run then Rest System changes that.

After each Dash, you take a Rest. And during the Rest, you stop trying to make any new changes.

Does that mean that you let go of the changes you just made in the Dash? The answer to that is neither yes or no. Instead, you just relax a bit.

If you've been strict about those changes during the Dash, then those changes will likely stick. For instance, if you started drinking more water during the previous Dash, then you'll likely keep drinking more water. Some days, you might miss the goals you'd set during the Dash, but that's ok.

In other words, you likely won't be as good as you were during the Dash. But that's fine. In fact, it's the whole point. You're giving your mind and body a rest, and even if you only keep 50% of the gains you made in the previous Dash, it's still 50% better than you were.

Habits and Imperfection

At first glance, this system can be a bit hard to accept. I know, because I've had many folks who were disbelievers at first.

But the way this system will help you most is that you will build small habits into your life that make you gradually healthier and healthier. Those changes will begin to add up, and you will begin to lose weight without even trying—often during the Rest periods as well.

And above all else, you will be able to keep going. After all, even if you crash and burn during a Dash period, all you need to do is to take a brief Rest and then start another Dash.

I've seen this work for countless people, and it can work for you.

A Quick and Easy Summary of the Run then Rest System

In case the above chapter wasn't clear enough, here is a quick recap of how the Run then Rest System works. Also, in the next Chapter, I have included a Quick Start Guide with a suggested set of Dashes and Rests, so that you don't need to create your own. That is where I recommend that you start.

Step 1: **Pick 1-3 changes to make to your diet/lifestyle (preferably from the set of Big Wins in this book).**

Step 2: **Commit to 1-2 months of making those changes.** (You choose exactly how long, but between 1 and 2 months.)

Step 3: **For those 1-2 months, be as strict as possible with those changes.** Track them every single day. Post a Calendar/Checklist where you can see it and physically check off the changes every day. Either make your own calendar or download the calendar from http://jeremyhendon.com/accidental-weight-loss-calendar.

Step 4: **After the 1-2 months, take a 1 month Rest.**

Step 5: **During the Rest, some of the changes will likely stick, but don't force it. Forget for this month about weight loss and focus on another area of your life.**

Step 6: **Start again with Step 1.** You can choose the same changes if you felt like they didn't stick, or you can choose new improvements to your diet/lifestyle.

Chapter 15

QUICK-START GUIDE

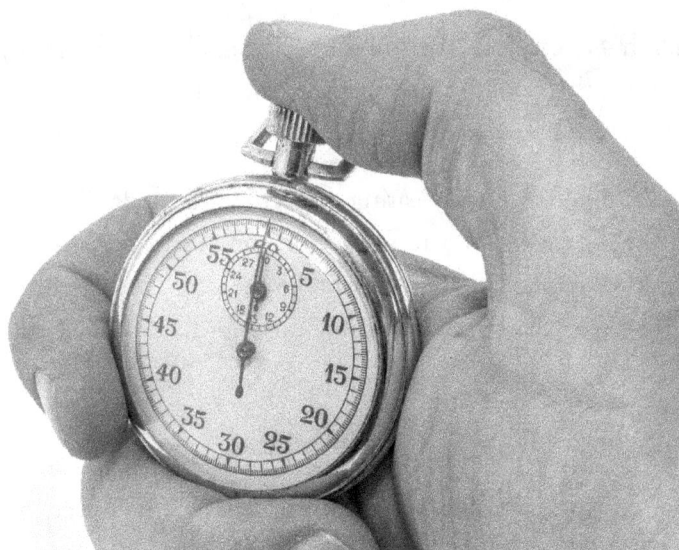

MUCH OF THIS book has been information. Information is important.

But nothing is more important than just getting started.

So in this chapter, I will show you an <u>exact step-by-step plan for applying the Run then Rest System for losing weight</u> (using the Big Wins I showed you in Part 2).

I've selected these particular Big Wins, and I've put them in this particular order because it's what works most often. Some of the Dashes might seem small or insignificant. That is the point.

If you can make these changes part of your life, then you'll be that much closer to having all the fundamentals in place for starting to accidentally and automatically lose weight. **Your body wants to be healthy, and often it's the small changes that allow your body to do so**.

Dash #1, in particular, might seem small and simple. But even while writing this book, I went back and did Dash #1 again, because I realized that these habits had slipped a little bit in my own life.

Also, if you're already eating a strict real-food or Paleo diet, then Dash #2 will be a bit of a refresher for you. You can skip this Dash if you want, but I encourage you to take the opportunity to revisit your diet and make it as strict as possible during this time.

Above All Else, Do Something

I want to help you lose weight. And I assume you want the same thing.

As you can probably tell, there are a lot of things you *might* need to change. Often, people get discouraged or overwhelmed, and then they don't do anything at all. That's the worst thing that can happen.

I've included this Quick-Start Guide to make it simpler to get started. This Quick-Start Guide tells you exactly what to do and when, so that you don't need to think about it at all if you don't want to.

If you don't want to start with this Quick-Start Guide, then feel free to implement the Big Wins into your own life however you feel is best. But remember that adding just 1-2 changes at a time to your life generally works best. Master those changes until they become automatic, and then layer another couple changes into your life.

In my own life, I have often tried to do too much all at once, and it has never turned out well. So take it slowly, master each change, and learn to permanently improve your life.

Quick Explanation

If you're ready to get started losing weight by accident, the Quick-Start Guide below is the best and easiest way to do it.

This guide is based on the Big Wins from Part 2 and on the Run then Rest approach from Chapter 14. And it will allow you to heal your body and lose weight automatically because it accomplishes the 8 Fundamental Principles from Chapter 4.

If you haven't read the rest of the book, that's OK. You can get started anyway. But I encourage you to read everything at some point, because your ability to understand what's happening with your body will make everything easier. You'll also understand why this Quick-Start Guide is organized the way that it is.

This is a Quick-Start Guide, but it lasts for 12 months. That sounds contradictory, but it's not. I'm giving you the fastest and best way to get started, but I want you to get permanent results. Take it one step at a time, and you'll be there before you know it.

You are welcome to start with any Dash that you want or to create your own. The schedule below is the one that I've found to work best for almost everybody. You might feel as though parts of it are too basic or not applicable to you, but that's almost never the case. Mastering the basics and fundamentals are exactly what will allow you to lose weight by accident and then keep it off for the rest of your life.

Finally, you can start on any day. I list the Dashes by month, but you could easily start on the 20th of a month and you'd simply end on the 20th of the following month.

The Quick-Start Guide

Prior to Starting:

1. Chapter 17 contains a Calendar/Checklist based on this Quick-Start Guide. Please either print out the calendar or tear it out of the book and put it up in your home where you will see it several times a day. Every day during a Dash, use the Calendar/Checklist to check off your progress, even if you "failed" that day.

2. Chapter 16 contains an exercise to get clear on your pain (this is the Big Win from Chapter 5). Set aside 45 minutes and do this exercise.

Month #1—Dash #1:

Implement Big Wins #2 and #3 from Chapter 6. In particular:

1. Every day, drink 1 glass of water immediately upon waking, and drink 1 glass of water immediately before every meal (including breakfast).

2. Every morning, eat at least 35 grams of protein at breakfast. (See Chapter 6 for examples.)

Month #2—Rest:

Relax and stop tracking the Big Wins from Dash #1. You will likely keep them to some degree, but it's also OK if they slip a bit.

Months #3-4—Dash #2:

Implement Big Win #1 from Chapter 6. In particular:

1. Eat zero processed sugar, gluten, dairy, or alcohol. Refer back to Chapter 6 for examples of these foods. Be 100% strict for these 2 months. If you need a sample meal plan, visit http://paleomagazine.com and download the free 4-week meal plan there—it's entirely free of highly inflammatory foods.

Month #5—Rest:

Relax and stop tracking the Big Win from Dash #2. By this time, you will certainly have noticed some positive (and perhaps amazing) changes in your body. Again, you will likely continue to eat fewer inflammatory foods, but don't worry if you slip a little bit.

Month #6—Dash #3:

Implement Big Wins #1 and #2 from Chapter 7. In particular:

1. Every day, walk at least 10,000 steps. Be very strict about this and find a way to get the steps every single day.

2. Do some type of resistance training 2 times per week. Refer back to Chapter 7 for examples or suggested routines.

Month #7—Rest:

By now, you've done a lot, so you should enjoy this rest. You will continue to move more and eat fewer inflammatory foods, but don't track it or worry about it.

Month #8—Dash #4:

Implement Big Win #1 from Chapter 8. In particular:

1. Every single day, be in bed in the dark for at least 9 hours. This is your only Big Win for this Dash, because it's harder than it sounds, so stay focused and be very strict.

Month #9- Rest:

The same as all of the Rests above.

Months #11-12—Dash #5:

For this Dash, you have a choice:

1. If your diet has not been very strict over the last few months, then do Dash #2 again and eliminate all processed sugar, gluten, alcohol, and dairy.

2. If your diet has been pretty good, then implement Big Win #1 from Chapter 12. Choose to fast for either (a) 16 hours every day or (b) 36 hours one time per week.

Where Do You Go From Here?

If you get through the Quick-Start Guide above, then chances are that you'll look and feel completely different than you did 12 months earlier. And your life and energy levels will be dramatically improved.

The best part is—by building habits through the Run then Rest approach, most of these habits will stick at least a little bit. That doesn't mean you'll be perfect or that you won't slip up, but every little bit of improvement will build on itself, and you'll lose more weight and feel better than ever.

Obviously, there are several Big Wins that are not included in this Quick-Start Guide. So if you get done and want to lose even more weight or feel even better, then start implementing the other Big Wins. In particular, the Big Wins from Chapters 9, 10, and 11 can make huge differences in your life. I think it's most important to have everything else in place first, but when you're ready, start adding those into your life through other Dashes.

I've created a complete Calendar/Checklist for you to use along with this Quick-Start Guide—you can download it from http://jeremyhendon. com/accidental-weight-loss-calendar. And in Chapter 16, I've included the exercise that you should do immediately.

I mention this in the Introduction and at the end of the book, but if you have any questions that aren't covered in this book, please reach out to me at jeremy@jeremyhendon.com. I love hearing from readers both in terms of what's working and what isn't.

Chapter 16

ONE THING TO DO IMMEDIATELY

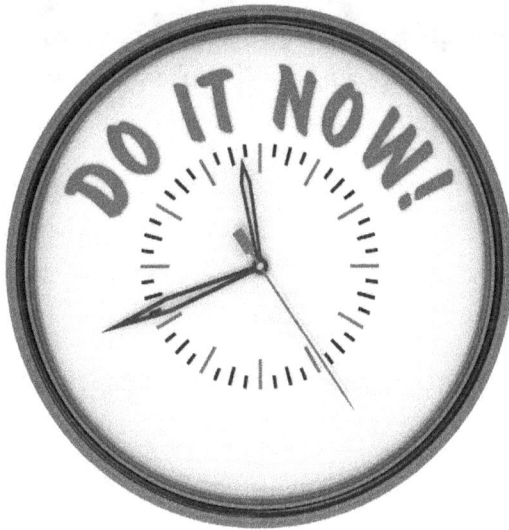

B EFORE YOU DO anything else from this book, I strongly suggest
that you complete the 5-part exercise in this chapter.

In just 30-45 minutes, this exercise will get you your first Big Win (get
clear on your pain from Chapter 5). You won't lose any weight in the

next 30–45 minutes, but the effects of this exercise will last for months or years.

But you must take this exercise seriously. I suggest finding a space where you'll be undisturbed for at least 45 minutes and where you can write, because you MUST write for this exercise—it won't work as well otherwise.

When you're ready, here's what to do . . .

Part #1: Write Down All the <u>Pleasure</u> You Get from <u>NOT Losing Weight</u>

This might sound like an odd question, because you think that not losing weight causes you pain. But if you're honest, you also get some benefits from not losing weight.

Maybe it means that you get to eat your favorite food or snack, you don't have to stress as much, or you get to keep living your same comfortable life. Maybe you don't need to buy new clothes. Be honest, because you definitely get something out of it.

Spend 5 minutes writing down on a sheet of paper all of the pleasures you can think of that come from not losing weight. Even if they seem small or silly, write them down.

What pleasure do you get from NOT losing weight?

_____

_____

_____

_____

_____

_____

_____

_____

_____

Part #2: Write Down All the <u>Pain</u> You Get from <u>Not Losing Weight</u>.

What is it costing you to not lose weight?

Do you feel uncomfortable with yourself? Is your health suffering? Do you have less energy to play a sport or spend time with family?

Really imagine all the pain that it's causing you RIGHT NOW, and spend 5 minutes writing it all down.

_____

_____

_____

_____

_____

_____

_____

_____

Part #3: Imagine Yourself <u>5 Years Older</u> Than You Are Today. <u>You Still Haven't Lost Any Weight</u>. How Will You Feel? What <u>Pain</u> Will That Cause You?

Picture yourself 5 years in the future and 5 years older. You still haven't lost any weight (or perhaps you've even gained some).

How does that make you feel? Are you angry, sad, depressed? What kind of pain is it causing you at that point? Has your health gotten worse? Do you feel even worse about who you are? Do you feel like you've wasted those 5 years?

Spend another 5 minutes and write down exactly how you'll feel and exactly what it's costing you and what kinds of pain it's causing in your life.

_____

_____

_____

_____

_____

_____

_____

_____

_____

_____

Part #4: Imagine Yourself <u>10 Years Older</u> Than You Are Today. <u>You STILL Haven't Lost Any Weight</u>. What <u>Pain</u> Do You Feel in That Situation?

You are 10 years older—another decade has passed between today and then. And you've chosen not to do what it takes to lose any weight. You still look and feel the same, just 10 years older.

How will that make you feel? Will you look back on those 10 years and wonder what happened? Will it make you feel a little sick in your stomach to think of the missed opportunity? Will you have the energy to excel at work or to spend quality time with your family?

Spend 5 minutes to write down how you'll feel after 10 years of not losing any weight and what pain it will be causing you.

At this point, you might think that you can skip this part of the exercise, since you've done it for now and for 5 years from now. But remember that this is important to you, and you need to get absolutely clear on the pain not achieving your goals will cost you.

_____

_____

_____

_____

_____

_____

_____

Part #5: Write Down all the <u>Pleasure</u> You'll Get By <u>Immediately Taking Action</u> to Lose Weight

If you started right now in a serious effort to lose weight, what sorts of pleasure will that bring you?

Will you feel proud of yourself? Will it make you feel like you're actually progressing and reclaiming part of your life? Perhaps it will give you more energy or make you feel a little bit happier.

Again, spend 5 minutes writing down all the pleasure you'll get out of taking immediate action to start losing weight.

_____

_____

_____

_____

_____

_____

_____

_____

_____

_____

_____

Finally . . .

Stop for a moment and think about staying overweight. Do you feel even more uncomfortable than you did before the exercise? You should, and if you don't, then it might help to do the exercise again with a little bit more intensity and emotional commitment.

There is no right or wrong way to do this exercise. And even though it's a Big Win, it won't provide you with endless motivation and willpower.

However, you should by now be MUCH clearer on just how much pain it's causing you to not lose weight, and how much pleasure you'll get from following through.

If, by chance, you don't feel that pain and pleasure, then losing weight might not be as important to you as you thought. That's perfectly fine, but it's better to know than not to know.

Chapter 17

CALENDAR/CHECKLIST

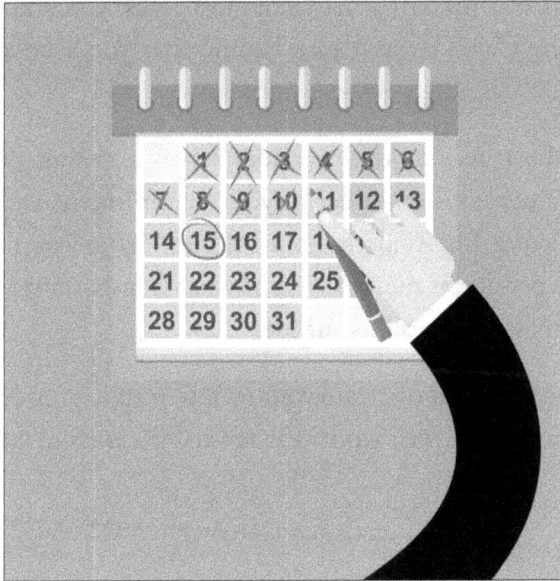

B ECAUSE I WANTED the Calendar/Checklist to be larger (so that you can post it in your home), I'm not including it in this book. Instead, you can download it for free and print it out at http://jeremyhendon.com/accidental-weight-loss-calendar.

The Calendar is a checklist for each Dash of the Quick-Start Guide. It has blanks for dates, so that you can start whenever makes sense for you.

Also, there is no checklist for the final Dash (#5), because that is an intermittent fasting Dash, and you may choose to (a) fast for 16 hours per day, (b) fast for 36 hours once per week, or (c) go back and redo Dash #2 if your diet has gotten a little out of control. Having a checklist for this Dash doesn't make sense because of the choices, but also because fasting is not necessarily an everyday occurrence.

The Calendar is simple. If you're like most folks, you'll be tempted to skip using the Calendar and just assume that you'll be able to keep track of it.

That might be true, but the Calendar serves a greater purpose. The Calendar is a constant reminder of your commitment and your focus on 1-2 particular Big Wins for that month. By seeing the Calendar several times per day, it reminds you of what is important and why you are making these changes in your life.

Please use the Calendar or create your own to post in your home. Either way, the effort will be well worth the reward in terms of weight loss.

PART IV

FREQUENTLY ASKED QUESTIONS & COMMON MISTAKES

Chapter 18

FREQUENTLY ASKED QUESTIONS

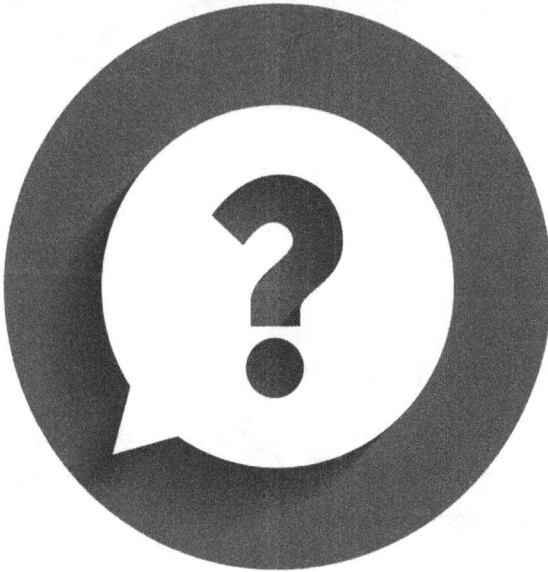

H ERE ARE SOME of the most common and frequent questions that I get asked about weight loss.

Question #1: How Often Should I Eat?

One of the Small Wins from Chapter 6 is to eat enough. It might surprise you, but I see a lot of people eat too little when they're trying to lose weight.

Obviously, gorging yourself is always going to be a problem, but in general, if you follow the Big Wins I've outlined in this book, you won't typically need to count calories or measure your food. It can be beneficial to do every once in a while for a week or so, but it's neither fun nor sustainable in the long run.

If you eat 2-3 meals per day, that's plenty. The great majority of research shows that eating fewer meals (rather than 4-6) is better for weight loss.

It doesn't really matter when you eat these meals, but most people find it easiest to stick to a normal breakfast, lunch, and dinner.

If you have thyroid or adrenal issues, then it often helps to eat a little bit more frequently. In those situations, 4-5 meals is fine, but make each meal a bit less food than you otherwise would.

Question #2: How Strict Should I Be?

The problem with most diets is that you can't keep it up for very long. You end up cheating and falling off of the diet. It's the reason that TV shows like The Biggest Loser don't have long-term success with their contestants.

The Run then Rest approach is designed to help you overcome this problem by building only the most important healthy habits into your life.

During a Dash, you should be as strict as possible. You're trying to build a new behavior into your life, and it helps to be strict for a little while. Plus, you're only doing it for 30-60 days, so it's possible to stay strict for that long. Also, being this strict will give you better results and keep you motivated.

During your Rests, though, you should relax and not worry about being strict. That doesn't mean that you should *try* to be unhealthy and lose the habits you've built. Just don't worry if they slip a little bit.

Question #3: What if I Cheat During a Dash?

You're going to slip up. It's only human. So not all of your Dashes (and likely not even your first one) are going to be perfect.

Don't worry about it. But do keep tracking yourself with the Calendar/ Checklist when you slip up. Tracking allows you to view it more objectively and not beat yourself up. In turn, that allows you to get back on track more quickly.

If a Dash goes very badly, then that's fine also. Just take a month of Rest and then try the Dash again.

Remember, you've probably spent most of your life building bad habits, gaining weight, and getting to the point you're at now. Losing weight, getting healthy, and building great habits might take a little bit of time.

You'll get great results in the meantime, but don't beat yourself up for not being perfect.

Question #4: What Should I Do During a Rest Period?

Relax and live your life like normal.

Don't track yourself, and don't worry about whether or not you get a little bit less healthy during this time. The point is to give your mind and body a rest so that you can stay motivated and also so that your body and mind have some time to get used to the changes you've made.

With that in mind, you shouldn't view the Rest as an opportunity to go crazy. Just approach it like normal. Some of your Big Wins will stick and others won't. That's fine.

Question #5: What if I Have an Illness or Special Conditions?

Because I don't know you personally (and also because I'm not a doctor or healthcare professional), I can't possibly give you specific advice for any particular condition. And if you have any sort of illness or medical issue, then please do make sure you clear everything with your doctor or healthcare professional.

With that in mind, I do want to mention a few specific situations where you might want to consider making other changes (or not making some of the changes I suggested).

1. **Diabetes or Insulin Resistance**. If you're a Type II Diabetic, Pre-Diabetic, or if you know that you're pretty insulin-resistant, then this is something you need to deal with. And generally, that means eating fewer carbs than you otherwise might. In these situations, your body simply can't properly deal with and metabolize carbs.

Many people who are diabetic or insulin resistant need to stay on low carb diets for a long time until their body recovers. If this is the case for you, be sure to eat plenty of vegetables and fermented foods to make sure that you feed your gut bacteria. If needed, you can also supplement with fibers like inulin, acacia, and/or psyllium husk.

2. **Adrenal Fatigue and/or Underactive Thyroid**. On the other side of the spectrum, if you have hypothyroid, adrenal fatigue, or similar issues, then you need to be eating more carbs in general. And you also potentially need to be eating more frequently.

For people not in this situation, I encourage eliminating all snacking, since that usually helps with weight loss. However, when you have thyroid and adrenal issues, eating more frequently can actually have a positive effect on weight loss.

3. **Autoimmune Disorders**. If you have any sort of autoimmune disorder (Graves', Hashimoto's, Addison's, Crohn's, etc.), then you almost certainly need to be on an AIP diet, which is a stricter form of Paleo. Your body is much more sensitive to a variety of foods, including eggs, nightshades, and other foods that are typically considered healthy.

In addition, getting tested (see Chapter 11) is extra important, because it's almost inevitable that your body will have pathogens and deficiencies. It's almost impossible to effectively treat an autoimmune disorder without getting tested.

Question #6: Should I Try Intermittent Fasting?

Intermittent Fasting usually works one of two ways. One way is to confine your eating to a block of time every day (say between 10am-

6pm), so that you don't eat for the other 16 hours of the day (6pm-10am). The other way is to simply fast for an entire day once per week.

From a research perspective, intermittent fasting shows some promise. And from a practical perspective, many people have lost weight through intermittent fasting.

So if you want to try it, I'm not going to discourage you.

However, here are a few things to take into consideration:

1. Don't try it unless you've incorporated most of the other Big Wins in this book (particularly Chapters 6, 7, & 8). If you're not eating well, or if you're sleeping too little, or anything else, then your body will be fairly stressed and inflamed. And if that's the case, then intermittent fasting is just going to add to the burden. On the other hand, if you're doing everything else well, then the temporary stress from intermittent fasting can work in your body's favor. The point is, don't try it until everything else is in place.

2. If you have hypothyroid or adrenal fatigue, intermittent fasting may make your situation worse. Your body will have trouble producing energy (because of too little T3 or too little cortisol), so be careful.

Question #7: What if I'm an Athlete?

If you're an athlete or just very active, then you likely already have most of the exercise habits incorporated into your life.

Everything else is going to stay the same, except for the fact that you need to make sure you eat enough food. That may require you keeping in some foods (such as white rice) to give you easy access to calories.

Otherwise, you probably need to sleep even more than average (most athletes do), and you might want to get tested for pathogens more regularly, since your body is under additional stress from your sport and more likely to play host to malicious micro-organisms.

Question #8: Should I Eat Low Carb or Low Fat?

Unless you're insulin-resistant (including diabetic), I recommend that you don't worry about either carbs or fat. Because you're cutting out all processed sugar and most grains and legumes, you're automatically going to eat fewer carbs than the average person.

But that's not the same as low carb. If you're measuring it, I suggest you get somewhere between 100-200 grams of carbs per day, although a little above or below that should be fine also.

In the end, though, I don't think it's necessary to measure. Just keep eating real food, keep avoiding all processed sugar, gluten, and dairy, and you'll be fine.

Chapter 19

COMMON MISTAKES

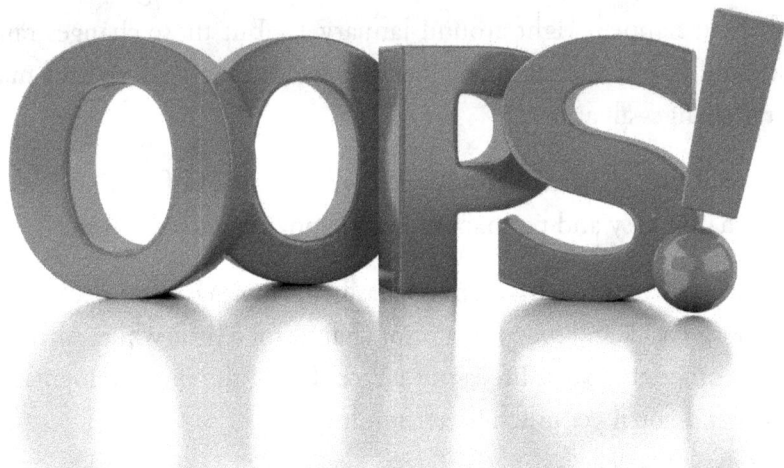

YOU'RE GOING TO make some mistakes. We all do.

But so long as you're aware of your mistakes, you'll be able to correct them as you go along, and they won't set you back very far.

In general, I see most people make the same mistakes over and over again, so I decided to list a few of the most common mistakes in this final chapter. Hopefully, as you're improving your diet and lifestyle, you'll occasionally think back to these mistakes and examine your own life to see if you've fallen into any of these traps.

Mistake #1: Doing Everything All At Once

This is the saddest mistake to make, because it means you're really serious about trying to lose weight and improve your health. But it also means that you're ignoring what's happened to you in the past.

We've all tried many times to make a bunch of changes in our life. Usually it happens right around January 1st. But those changes rarely last, and one of the reasons is because we assume that we can make thirty changes all at once.

Don't fall into that temptation. Take your time and focus on making each change easy and permanent before moving onto the next.

Even with this approach, you may still slip up, but that's fine, because you can just go back and focus on a prior change for a little while. Although it feels otherwise, your life is not a race. Enjoy the improvements you make, and you'll get much better results.

Mistake #2: Not Resting

Once you start losing weight and feeling better, it's going to be tempting to just keep going. You'll get through your first Dash, you'll get a couple Big Wins under your belt, and you'll imagine how great it will be to lose even more weight.

But that's a huge mistake.

Remember that your body and brain can't keep going forever. You've got limited willpower, and your body needs time to adjust—both physically and psychologically.

When you first start a Rest, you'll probably be scared that you'll lose all of the progress you made during a Dash. But rest assured that you won't. You might lose a little bit of progress, but over the long-run, it's worth it, because you'll be able to keep going, keep getting more Big Wins, and keep losing more weight.

Plus, the Rests will allow you to have more fun, enjoy your life more, and still make progress.

Mistake #3: Not Focusing on Big Wins

So often, I see somebody get started with losing weight, and then a few weeks later, they'll tell me how they've stalled or have fallen off the wagon.

Typically, when I ask them what went wrong, they dodge the question at first. But once I get the answer out of them, it's always that they got distracted with something else. Sometimes they get distracted with inevitable life situations like illness or work.

But just as often, they got distracted by trying something else they heard about that might help them lose weight or get healthier.

I'm sure you can relate. You probably have friends or family who tell you about everything they hear on the news or everything they try themselves. And sometimes—mostly by coincidence—they'll get some good results for a short time.

And you suddenly feel like you're missing out. You think that you also need to try whatever they're trying because you're not losing weight fast enough.

Don't fall for it. The Big Wins I've shown you in this book are 99% of what you need in order to have an amazing body and amazing health. While it's likely that other technology or tricks will come along to make things even better and easier, the Big Wins will always be the foundation that you need for accidental weight loss.

Focus on the Big Wins and don't sweat the small stuff.

Mistake #4: Assuming You Only Need to Do One Thing

Sometimes I'll coach somebody on weight loss or on improving their health, and I'll mention a few different things to them. Almost always, they'll latch onto one of the things I said and get really excited about making that one change.

Chances are, you need to make quite a few changes. That can be daunting at first, but it's also empowering. Because it means that all the other changes you make aren't useless—they're just steps along the road to better health and weight loss.

In the Quick-Start Guide alone, there are 7 Big Wins. Hopefully, you're already incorporating some of those changes into your life, but the reason I've listed those actions is because any one of them could be holding you back.

Don't assume that any one change is going to make all the difference. It's usually a combination of multiple changes.

Mistake #5: Doing Nothing

The most common thing that happens when somebody buys a book like this one is that they do nothing.

My job is to make the path as simple and clear as possible for you to get started (and to show you the path most likely to lead to success). Unfortunately, that's all I can do. You must take the action yourself.

I hope you've enjoyed this book and found it enlightening, but I really hope that you take my suggestions and use them in your own life. As I've mentioned several times, it's still going to be hard at points, but pretty much everything in life worth getting takes a little bit of work.

Mistake #6: Underestimating Stress

Some people know how stressed they are, but most of us assume that we're less stressed than is actually the case.

I didn't include any of the Big or Small Wins from Chapter 10 in the Quick-Start Guide. But that doesn't mean they don't matter.

And at some point, you'll need to deal with the stress in your life.

Even if you don't think you're very stressed, implement the Chapter 10 suggestions into your life anyway. Walk more. Get outside. Meditate. And start to deal with incongruities in your life.

Those are all things that will make you happier even if you're not that stressed. But the more likely outcome is that you'll start to realize how stressed you were, you'll start to deal with it, and you'll start to lose more weight.

Mistake #7: Assuming You're Different

To a degree, all of our bodies are different. We have slightly different genetics, slightly different circumstances, and slightly different problems.

But in the end, 99.99% is the same. And that means you need to start with all the same actions.

Along the way, you're going to learn a lot about your body and what affects you more or less than other people, but don't assume that gluten, lack of sleep, or stress don't affect you. They affect 100% of humans, just to varying degrees and in different ways.

Like Wilbur and Orville Wright, weight loss is all about doing all the right things first and then having the rest of the pieces fall into place.

REFERENCES

Introduction

1. http://www.wright-brothers.org/History_Wing/Wright_ Story/Career_Choices/Printing_&_Popcorn/Printing_&_ Popcorn.htm

Chapter 4

1. https://www.researchgate.net/profile/Ahmad_Aljada/ publication/8940222_Inflammation_The_link_ between_insulin_resistance_obesity_and_diabetes/ links/564c89d308aeab8ed5e9f2ac.pdf

2. http://www.jle.com/download/ecn-268297- recent_advances_in_the_relationship_between_ obesity_inflammation_and_insulin_resistance-- V5jLyX8AAQEAABlaUD8AAAAJ-a.pdf

3. http://www.nature.com/nm/journal/v11/n2/full/nm1185. html

4. http://content.onlinejacc.org/article. aspx?articleid=1139265

5. http://citeseerx.ist.psu.edu/viewdoc/download?doi=10.1.1.665.774&rep=rep1&type=pdf

6. http://www.wageningenacademic.com/doi/abs/10.3920/BM2013.006

7. http://www.tandfonline.com/doi/abs/10.1080/07315724.2007.10719658

8. http://www.healthybeveragesinchildcare.org/qa/DAnci.2006.NutrtionInClinicalCare.pdf

9. http://www.ncbi.nlm.nih.gov/pmc/articles/PMC1216967/pdf/8611144.pdf

Chapter 6

1. 500mL before meals reduces energy intake by 13%—http://www.ncbi.nlm.nih.gov/pubmed/18589036

2. Pre-meal water reduces energy intake: http://www.ncbi.nlm.nih.gov/pubmed/17228036

3. Pre-meal water significantly increases weight loss: http://www.ncbi.nlm.nih.gov/pubmed/19661958

4. Water increases energy burning for a short while after drinking: http://press.endocrine.org/doi/full/10.1210/jc.2006-1438

5. Water increases calories burned by up to 30%: http://www.ncbi.nlm.nih.gov/pubmed/14671205

6. Dehydration significantly impacts brain function, even if you're only slightly dehydrated: http://www.tandfonline.com/doi/abs/10.1080/07315724.2007.10719658

7. 1-2% dehydration (by bodyweight) can lead to cognitive decline: http://www.healthybeveragesinchildcare.org/qa/DAnci.2006.NutrtionInClinicalCare.pdf

8. Hydrations affects cell metabolism and gene expression: http://www.ncbi.nlm.nih.gov/pmc/articles/PMC1216967/pdf/8611144.pdf

9. Protein in Morning leads to reduced appetite and reduced feeding: http://www.nature.com/ijo/journal/v34/n7/full/ijo20103a.html

10. Protein (35g+) in morning improves blood-sugar control: http://www.nature.com/ijo/journal/v39/n9/full/ijo2015101a.html

11. Protein-rich breakfast reduces hunger and calorie-intake: http://www.pork.org/wp-content/uploads/2015/09/leidy-2015-obesity-2.pdf

12. High protein in morning leads to less snacking later, as well as total calorie intake: http://ajcn.nutrition.org/content/97/4/677.long?utm_source=youtube&utm_medium=social&utm_co__%253Futm_source=youtube&utm_co__?utm_source=youtube&utm_co__

Chapter 12

1. Fasting Leads to Autophagy: http://www.ncbi.nlm.nih. gov/pubmed/21106691

2. IF Leads to Longer Lifespan: http://openwritings. net/sites/default/files/excerpt/files/J.%20Nutr.-1946-Carlson-363-75.pdf

3. IF decreases risk of both cancer and cardiovascular disease: http://ajcn.nutrition.org/content/86/1/7.full

4. IF causes increase in growth hormone: http://www.ncbi. nlm.nih.gov/ pubmed?Db=pubmed&Cmd=ShowDetail View&TermToSearch=1548337&ordinalpos=9&itool= EntrezSystem2.PEntrez.Pubmed.Pubmed_ResultsPanel. Pubmed_RVDocSum

5. IF increases brain performance: http://www.ncbi.nlm.nih. gov/pubmed/12558961